READY, SET, ACHIEVE!

READY,
SET,
ACHIEVE!

A Guide to Taking Charge of Your Life,
Creating Balance and Achieving Your Goals

YURI DIOGENES
JODI MILLER

New York

READY, SET, ACHIEVE!

A Guide to Taking Charge of Your Life,

Creating Balance and Achieving Your Goals

© 2016 **YURI DIOGENES & JODI MILLER**.

Published in New York, New York, by Morgan James Publishing. Morgan James and The Entrepreneurial Publisher are trademarks of Morgan James, LLC.
www.MorganJamesPublishing.com

The Morgan James Speakers Group can bring authors to your live event. For more information or to book an event visit The Morgan James Speakers Group at www.TheMorganJamesSpeakersGroup.com.

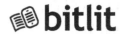

A **free** eBook edition is available with the purchase of this print book.

CLEARLY PRINT YOUR NAME ABOVE IN UPPER CASE

Instructions to claim your free eBook edition:
1. Download the BitLit app for Android or iOS
2. Write your name in **UPPER CASE** on the line
3. Use the BitLit app to submit a photo
4. Download your eBook to any device

ISBN 978-1-63047-589-5 paperback
ISBN 978-1-63047-590-1 eBook
Library of Congress Control Number:
2015937315

Cover Design by:
Rachel Lopez
www.r2cdesign.com

Interior Design by:
Bonnie Bushman
bonnie@caboodlegraphics.com

In an effort to support local communities and raise awareness and funds, Morgan James Publishing donates a percentage of all book sales for the life of each book to Habitat for Humanity Peninsula and Greater Williamsburg

Get involved today, visit
www.MorganJamesBuilds.com

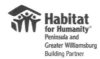

Habitat
for Humanity®
Peninsula and
Greater Williamsburg
Building Partner

TABLE OF CONTENTS

ACKNOWLEDGEMENTS

Yuri Diogenes

First and foremost, I would not be able to accomplish everything that I did without the true blessing of God; I give him all the credits for my success. I would like to thank my wife and daughters for their extreme support throughout my entire journey of getting this better version of me, Alexsandra, Yanne and Ysis I love you all! My great co-author and friend Jodi Miller, thanks for your friendship, guidance and expertise; it was an honor working with you on this project. To Jim Rowe for believing in this project and supporting us to make this happen. To my former coach and friend, Greg McCoy, I learned a lot from you and I will never be able to express my gratitude for everything you did to me, thank you buddy. To my current coach and friend, Jeff Dwelle, thank you for stepping up in the right time and believe in my potential, thanks for your true friendship. To all trainers and friends from Destination, Dallas: thanks for your inspiration and for making a difference. To all my team mates from Dwelle Athletics, thanks for your support, keep rocking!

I may have tons of more people to thank, but I will summarize saying: for all of you that were following this journey, hitting "like" on every progress that I posted on Facebook, motivating me with your words: THANK YOU! Thanks Morgan James Publishing Team for giving us the opportunity to have this book published.

Jodi Leigh Miller

My first words of gratitude go to my grandparents and parents for surrounding me with books, for feeding my addiction to reading by taking me to the library as often as I liked, for saving the stories I wrote—even way back in elementary school—and showing them to me while exclaiming, "we always knew you would write!", and for asking me constantly, "did you ever finish that story?". I also really need to thank my parents for not having any other children. As an only child—and an only grandchild—I grew up with a vivid imagination and a voracious love for words, and both of these qualities may have been squashed if other siblings existed to interrupt my daydreams and make believe efforts.

I need to thank my four high school English teachers: Ms. Pearson, Ms. Johnson, Ms. Jones, and Ms. Foster. My writing flourished under their guidance, and I actually became a high school English teacher because of these four wonderful, intelligent, and patient women.

I have extensive gratitude to my former colleagues in and my experience at the Texas Teaching Fellows, an affiliate of The New Teacher Project. So much of what I learned while I served as an instructional leader for this non-profit organization in terms of how to be an excellent manager and how to teach teachers soundly applies to motivating people to meet their own lifestyle and fitness goals. I definitely would not be who I am today without my years of experience there.

I also have utmost thanks for both of my powerlifting coaches—DJ and Dennis—and for all of the contest prep coaches I have had throughout my 15 years of competing: Brion Jackson, Jason English, Eric Jones, Mike Davies, Pete Grubbs, Jeremy Minihan, John Meadows, Jeff Dwelle. I am who I am as a competitor and coach today because of each one of these individuals. I wouldn't be able to describe step-by-step plans of action in the fitness industry without the vast information each one of these individuals provided to me.

I especially have to say thank you to Greg McCoy for opening his gym doors to me: first as a powerlifter and bodybuilder all the way back in 2010, then as a personal trainer and competition posing coach, and finally as a writer and editor. Greg has been the bridge that connected Yuri and me, which ultimately made this book a possibility. Along those same lines, I need to say thank you to the …destination family. I have yearned and earned and learned so much inside of this gym and plan to continue to do all three of those things long after this book is published. And thank you to Yuri Diogenes, for sharing this opportunity with me and bringing me on as a co-author and editor, for trusting my talent, and for providing utmost patience and understanding during an eventful year. I learned so much with him on this project. Additionally, thank you to former personal training client, Jim Rowe, for believing in this project and supporting us in this venture.

I dedicate this book to my grandparents, Mama Delle and Papa Sid. I know they are always smiling down on me. They live on through me.

FOREWORD

I have a tremendous amount of respect and admiration for both of these authors. I feel privileged to have both personal and professional relationships with both of them and couldn't be happier to be involved in the completion of "Achieve Your Best". The first time I spoke to Yuri about this project we were planning to write the book together. Due to my own goals, and complex set of life balances, I made a tough choice not to work on this book with him. This was very hard decision for me because authoring a book does happen to be on one of my "lists" that you'll read about near the end of this book. However having read this book I think it's safe to say that this is a great example of "everything happens for a reason." I enjoyed this book so much, and I'm glad that these two great people could come together and share their formulas for success and happiness to readers around the world.

I'll never forget meeting Yuri for the first time. I had just gotten off stage at the 2011 NPC Heart of Texas where I had competed and coached a number of clients, including one of Yuri's good friends. Yuri came up to me and expressed his interest in training and said that he would be contacting me soon. I have trained hundreds of athletes personally, and having owned a highly competitive gym for the last 7 years, I have seen thousands of athletes pursue a wide range of fitness goals. I have always had a tough habit of investing in people emotionally, which often times can be frustrating when you see people stray from their goals. Yuri on the other hand, sometimes I thought I should have been paying him instead of the other way around. He would systematically attack his goals time after time, and I would get so excited every time we would check in and he would literally crush the goal he set out for. I gained so much inspiration and energy from Yuri; I truly felt like the privilege was on my side. I have never had a client that was so methodical about their approach to goal setting and planning; sometimes even though I was the one writing the plans, I would have to make sure I was staying ahead of him! If there was ever someone I knew that should write a blueprint to achieving your best it should be Yuri. You don't really see someone's character until you see him or her deal with adversity though. We hit a few sticking points on Yuri's journey to his new life and new body. One time I'll never forget I hadn't heard from Yuri in a while and he called me talking about pushing back his bodybuilding goals and trying to do a long distance bicycle race. I told him jokingly, "Yuri, you're crazy!" It didn't take long to talk Yuri out of his detour into bicycle racing but I think about that not as a moment of weakness but of someone so motivated to achieve his best he was willing to do just about anything to find the best Yuri he knew he was capable of. Fast forward to the achievement of his goal of competing in a bodybuilding contest: Yuri stepped on stage with practically no body fat left and a physique that the Greeks would have deemed worthy of a statue. His transformation was like nothing I had ever seen. Most people that are in the condition that Yuri was in when his life was consumed by his career are lucky to lose enough weight to see their toes again, but Yuri lost ALL of his body fat. Following the exact steps he lays out in this book, he was able to take his body from one extreme to the other and manage an overall life balance through the process. Achieving a high level of career success in a country and a language that are not your own, raising a wonderful family, and transforming your body from obesity to competitive bodybuilding standards does not happen by accident. Find a quiet place and take a chance to learn from someone that talks the talk and walks the walk.

The moment in my relationship with Jodi that defines her is a powerlifting meet our gym hosted in 2013. I had never seen Jodi compete before but I was anticipating her performance on the platform. When she got to the deadlift portion of the meet, she had a look in her eyes that I can't really describe. I didn't doubt for one second that she was going to lift whatever was in front of her. We could've welded the weight to the floor and she probably would've ripped some of our gym's foundation up with the bar. I had a ton of respect for Jodi already, coming from a corporate career and making a leap of faith into a passion based career of fitness. She obviously wasn't scared of big challenges. But watching her lift that day, I saw some mettle in her that really inspired me. That same mettle with an educational and personal touch is also what makes all of her clients fall in love with her as a trainer and the results that she can create in them both on and off the gym floor.

I hope those of you reading this book, will read it and keep it close to you, almost like a manual, as you pursue your own journey into being your best.

Sincerely,
Greg McCoy
Co-Owner/General Manager
…destination Dallas, Texas Gym

Chapter 1

IT'S TIME TO CHANGE!

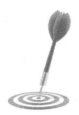

Introduction

Every time I watch the beginning to a Dreamworks production, I wonder what life would be like if we really could climb up to the moon, settle into the crook of it with our legs dangling, attach bait to a fishing line, and swing far and wide to catch our dreams. Would we have the same appreciation for our achievements if it were that simple? I doubt it.

But the starting line of reaching our goals actually does exist in a farfetched, fairy tale-like world. We typically see another person doing something we wish to do, or we experience a change in our lives that sparks our desire to move to a different rung on the life ladder. Whatever it is that initiates the spark,

1

that ember is a very necessary part to our ability to grab a fishing pole, hook bait upon the line, and swing with all of our might to catch the big one.

The thing is, we cannot simply grab that pole and catch our metaphorical fish in any body of water. We have to determine what type of fish we wish to catch, where the best place is to catch such a fish, what type of bait will attract that variety of fish, and what we will do should changes in weather, lake levels, or boat maintenance change. This means that while achievement of goals begins in the recesses of our imagination, order and organization must exist if we expect to actually attain said goals with any measure of success. This chapter will delve into how we can go about doing exactly that.

Setting a Winning Goal

We could begin this section with a discussion of desire, but in all honesty, desire is the easiest part of this whole process. So instead, let's jump straight into the deep end and examine how to set a goal. One word sums up this process well: SMART.

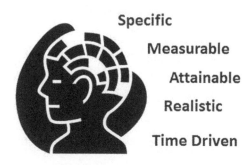

Specific

Measurable

Attainable

Realistic

Time Driven

Figure 1-1: SMART

The SMART acronym, as shown in Figure 1-1 displays the following five necessary components to successful goal setting:

1. **A goal must be specific.**

   If a goal is vague, the outcome will be blurry and fuzzy as well. If we wish to have crisp, sharp, precise changes in our lives, then our goals must have the same clarity. We cannot simply state we wish to lose weight and expect a considerable shift in our appearance. We must narrow the focus of our goal. Is this one pound or 20 pounds? Is it fat we wish to lose or muscle? Do we care from where we lose the weight, or are we focused on our derrieres? Do we have a lifetime to lose this weight, or are we trying to fit into a bikini or bathing trunks for a summer vacation? When we add details to the goal at hand, we see our eventual results better and can plan a precise path to our change more adequately and appropriately.

2. **A goal must be measurable.**

   This sounds redundant to the "specific" portion of the SMART acronym, but this is where a little mathematics comes into play: numbers and percentages. We will stick with the losing weight scenario to explain this since ultimately this book is focused on your ability to transform your body in today's society. What if you set a goal to lose 20 pounds? That seems specific enough, right? But how will you measure this goal of 20 pounds? Will you weigh yourself at the end of your designated time for achieving this goal? What if you are building muscle and don't lose 20 pounds but actually look better than you did if you only lost 20 pounds of fat and didn't gain an ounce of muscle? Would that mean you failed? No. So determining a specific measure for this weight-loss goal is extremely important to ensure you are attaining the exact change you wish to achieve. You might instead have a goal of fitting into a size-six bikini or a 32-waistline for men's swim trunks and seeing the outline of your obliques when that time comes. Now, with a measurable element in hand, it is okay if you do not quite reach a 20-pound weight loss since you would presumably gain muscle while you simultaneously work towards this overall goal. As you can see, we have taken a specific goal and added a measuring tape to it.

3. **A goal must be aligned to one's life or attainable with one's resources and time allotment.**

The Biggest Loser and other weight-loss reality shows often depict massive weight loss achievements. We are talking 100-pounds or more in a very short span of time. What we forget when we talk about these shows the next day around the proverbial water cooler at work is that the contestants on these shows are spending upwards of six to eight hours per day sweating, grunting, running, lifting and also have access to very vocal, passionate coaches who watch their every move like a hawk waiting for road kill. Most of us don't have this luxury of time, amount of energy, or monetary expenditure; thus setting a goal to lose 100 pounds in less than six months would not only set us up for failure but would be a truly unhealthy, rapid result in the span of our lives. So after adding specificity and measurement to our goal, we need to assess our budget, our schedules, the people with whom we share our lives, our other goals (since we can and should attain more than one goal at a time), and many other influences in order to determine if we can reasonably insert this goal into our lives without driving ourselves insane in the process.

4. **A goal must be realistic.**

   There is a distinct difference between a dream and a goal. Winning the lottery fits into the category of a dream because it is dependent upon so many factors outside of our control. No matter how diligent we are, we may never achieve the correct selection of winning numbers. In contrast, a goal is typically chosen based upon one's time, resources, and capabilities. And these are the factors that determine whether the goal is truly realistic. If I am a size 12, can I realistically fit into a size-four bathing suit within the next two months without causing damage to my metabolism? Additionally, do I have a gym membership? Do I have the funds for a personal trainer? What is my work schedule like? Is my partner someone who is understanding and supportive, or will I experience a hint of sabotage and jealousy that might slow down my progress? Is a size four even the right size for my body type? Maybe I should give myself six months to reach this goal rather than just two months. And maybe I should alter this goal to fitting into a size six pair of jeans by the fall months rather than a size-four bathing suit by the summer months. This way, I give myself a fighting chance to capture this goal instead of setting myself up for failure before I've even put bait onto my fishing line.

5. **A goal must be time driven.**

Have you ever had a boss or a friend or a significant other ask you to do a task or chore and simply told you, "as soon as you can"? Did you do it right away? Or did it get buried in a pile of other "as soon as you can" tasks while those with specific deadlines took priority? There is something about a specific date looming in front of us that gets our blood moving, our brains firing off, and our bodies working. Our goals are no different. If you simply tell yourself, "I want to fit into a size-six bikini," and you are at a Fourth of July dinner bash with your friends, you are less likely to pass on that cheesecake for dessert than if you have a goal of fitting into that same size-six bikini by July 31st. Putting your goal into a time capsule provides more insurance on the completion of the goal as well as allows for opportunities to set benchmarks along the way to measure your rate of success towards your goal.

Planning to Win

Typically, it is quite hard to give someone a task with minimal instructions or little direction and say, "just do it." Not everyone lives his or her life like a Nike commercial. Additionally so many in this day and age are too caught up in the mundane tasks of moving from one auto-pilot motion to the next without delving into how a particular action in present time affects the big picture. But this thought process does not work from a company perspective. Now, you might think, "Wait a minute; I'm not a company. What are you talking about? I'm a person, an individual." Well, in actuality you are your own company, and you are the CEO of it. You need structure and organization in your life; you have to pay yourself and pay others who render services to and for you; you have stocks in relationships, health, possessions; you have a career path, and you act as a guide for others who wish to follow in your footsteps. As a result, drafting a plan to achieve, improve, excel, and win becomes necessary when building the infrastructure of your future and the future of those who surround you (significant other, children, parents, friends, and others who provide value and meaning into your company, your world).

Remembering we have our SMART goal in place, let us examine how to draft the plan to achieve that very goal.

- Step One – Write a checklist of needs and wants.
- Step Two – Determine HWH (How, Why and How): How your goal may affect you and your surroundings, who and what will be affected, and how you can mitigate those effects.
- Step Three – Create a chronological timeline, utilizing backwards planning and inserting benchmark measures—or short-term goals—that propel forward motion towards your long-term goal.

Step One

Let us dig into the first step of planning to win, which is writing a checklist of elements that affect your achievement of your goal. If your goal is to lose three inches around your waist while increasing your strength by at least 10% in the next three months, you have to first determine the resources—tangible and intangible—you will need in your plan of action toward this goal. Basically, this is a list of items you should consider before you ever step foot onto your path of self-improvement. Below is an example of this list:

- Do I need a nutritional plan?
  - ▲ Do I need to hire someone, or can I determine on my own the caloric intake and macronutrients I need for healthy and sustainable weight loss/ muscle gain?
    - ○ If I need to hire someone, who is a reputable nutritionist or coach?
      - ★ What qualities am I looking for in this person?
      - ★ What expenditure am I willing to allocate to this person?
    - ○ If I can do it myself, what resources do I need?
      - ★ Software
      - ★ Books for research
      - ★ Website articles and forums
  - ▲ How much will following a specific plan cost?
  - ▲ What do I need to buy and do I have access to those items in my area?

- ▲ How many trips to the store will I need to make per week?
- ▲ How many meals a day will I need to prepare, and what is the time factor involved?
- ▲ Will my job allow my frequent eating?
- ▲ How will I pack my food if I am gone from the house for several hours?
- ▲ Are there any upcoming trips that may be affected by this food plan?
- • Do I need a training program?
  - ▲ How can I get this training program?
    - ○ Should I hire a personal trainer?
      - ★ How much am I willing to spend on a personal trainer or coach?
      - ★ What qualifications and experience do I wish for this trainer/coach to have?
      - ★ How often will I need to see this trainer?
    - ○ Can I get an online program, and from where on the Internet would I find one?
      - ★ How effective would this online program be for me? Will I really stick with it when I have little to no accountability? What are the pros and cons compared to hiring a trainer or coach?
  - ▲ Should I do more cardio or weight lifting? For how long? Which exercises do I do? Which equipment should I use?
  - ▲ How much time a day should I spend exercising?

- Do I need a gym membership?
  - ▲ If I am hiring a trainer, is the trainer at my current gym or at a different gym?
  - ▲ Where is the gym in location to my work/home commute?
  - ▲ If I travel for my job, do I have access to this gym franchise or another gym in the cities/states to which I'm traveling?
  - ▲ What does my company or boss offer in terms of monies for gym memberships?
- Do I have appropriate gym clothes? Tennis shoes?
- How many hours of rest do I need?
  - ▲ Do I need to sleep more?
    - ○ Will my job and family life allow for that?
  - ▲ Can I keep my stress level to a minimum?
    - ○ Will working out help or hinder that?
- Who is my support group?
  - ▲ Parents, friends, siblings, significant other? (Write a list of names.)
  - ▲ Would anyone object or feel uncomfortable by me bettering myself?
    - ○ Who?
    - ○ How will I deal with that negativity and keep it from affecting my path to success?

Of course, these are only sample questions that we initially suggest to bring to the surface, obtain the answers, and create a guided action plan based upon those answers. You may have more questions that rise up as you work your way through your checklist and even as you begin digging into your plan. Later on in this chapter, we will examine the need for flexibility, which is based upon a willingness to add, change, delete, and grow as the need arises, especially as smaller plans hatch out of the bigger picture. For example, you have a broad plan for losing three inches around the waist, which includes nutrition, working out, relying on your support group. Within that broad plan, you will also have a nutritional plan that has specific bullet points to follow, and you will have a training program that has specific step-by-step actions to follow. The diagram below demonstrates this plan-within-a-plan idea:

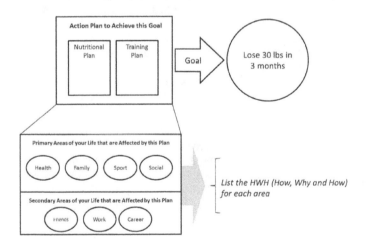

Figure 1-2: Components of HWH

Step Two
Now that you have a checklist of questions to answer and steps to take that will drive you towards your goal, you are now

ready for step two of the planning-to-win process. This involves concrete identification of areas and people in your life that will be affected by your journey towards your goal and is done by completing an HWH chart, seen in the table that it follows.

1. How your goal may affect you and your surroundings
2. Who and what will be affected
3. How you can mitigate those effects

Below is an example of how to use an HWH chart:

Area	How it will affect?	Who and why it will affect?	How can I mitigate the effect(s)?
Family	I might have to bypass some family events in the beginning of the program.	I might need to bypass the events because I will be depleted and have low energy level as well as time constraints. My children may be affected because they might have fewer opportunities of free time with me.	I might want to set the expectation[1] with my family that this might happen in the beginning but once I condition myself to this new regime I should be back. I might plan for shorter spells of time with my children throughout the week, like reading bedtime stories or drinking coffee with them while they eat their breakfast before school.

---

1   Setting expectations for everyone who is directly or indirectly involved in your pathway to change is a great strategy to communicate what might happen. Sometimes working as a hermit in which only you are aware of consequences can cause stressful situations. Be transparent

Social	I won't be able to go out and socialize with co-workers and friends.	My diet will be very strict and the places that we usually go just have junk food or take place during happy hour, which is a prime training time for me.	I need to schedule my "treat" meals[2] to match with those social meetings so that I can eat and enjoy the time with family and friends.
			I need to prepare my food in advance and bring it in plastic containers or call a restaurant to see if I can request specific foods and portions to fit my needs.
			I may work with my significant other to plan for a couple of get-togethers at our house in order to ensure the food I need is readily available in the quantities my meal plan requires.

As you can see, completing the HWH table is not that complicated and may even be a soothing or motivating mental exercise. As time passes, you will have this matrix memorized and may not even need paper or a computer to physically fill it in, though seeing the challenges and solutions in black and white often helps us to adhere to a plan. In addition, new challenges may arise and others may stay the same or even

---

and communicate with people who are in the areas that will be directly affected.

2   Read Chapter 3 of this book for more information about "treat" meals (also known as "cheat" meals or even "refeeds") and why it is important to have these included in your nutrition plan.

disappear, so please remember that this matrix should be considered dynamic—flexible and ever-changing—rather than static.

Step Three

A major part of planning to win involves the creation of a timeline and benchmarks that allow you to measure your timely success towards reaching your goal. You might think that you begin this timeline at the starting line, but in actuality it should be designed in a backwards fashion, from the finish line. Planning a vacation or trip is a perfect example of how backwards design works. If we wish to travel from Dallas to Las Vegas, we need to know the end date in order to determine how long we have to travel from our starting city to the final destination. We can then determine our means of transportation, what we wish to do in Las Vegas, when those particular shows or events are occurring

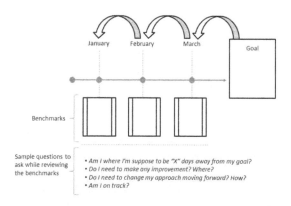

Figure 1-3: Checkpoints along the way

and accepting reservations, which hotels have available rooms, etc. Once we know these answers, we can then look for a departing flight or choose a starting driving date and time that will allow us to reach Las Vegas. Returning to our weight-loss goal, if we know that we wish to meet this goal by August 31st, then we are better able to work backwards from that point and know how far out to begin working towards this goal.

Timeline Towards My Weight Loss Goal

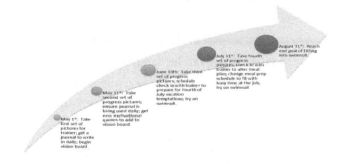

Figure 1-4: Celebrate major milestones in your journey

While Figure 1-3 shows the actual benchmarks that are set at specific dates to ensure the goal will be reached by the set date, Figure 1-4 shows how to work your way backwards from the end goal to the starting point, create specific questions, and set up benchmarks to track your progress in a measurable manner. Some of these benchmarks include checking in with the trainer, taking progress pictures, trying on the swimsuit, making alterations to the meal plan, re-examining a meal prep schedule, preparing for a vacation while still maintaining healthy eating habits, and gearing up for a busy time at work while not falling off the wagon. By stating a specific date, looking backwards to when the project should begin (as Figure 1-3 demonstrates), and moving forward to implement concrete action steps (as Figure 1-4 demonstrates), success will be attained.

But please note that once you complete these three steps, the planning process does not end there. Some or all of these steps may need to revisited—and not necessarily in the order in which we provided them. Reviewing a certain step, returning to a previous juncture, and relaxing in order to catch one's breath and remain sane are all part of the process. So be prepared to re-assess your situation often and be flexible should circumstances change or one area of your journey become more challenging than you originally imagined. This will allow you to remain proactive in making appropriate changes. It will also prevent you from punishing yourself or slipping in your self-esteem should you miss meeting a benchmark since you will be able to react with conviction rather than impulse. Again, remain pliable and flexible in your solutions, and you will not break when storms bend your branches.

The "No Excuses" Rule

No matter how well you plan, it is oftentimes still easier to fail than succeed. Notice we didn't say, "better." We just said, "easier." The path to failure is often laden with excuses that carry a great deal of thought process but little action. The first of several "One on One with the Author" anecdotes delves into a prime example of this.

One on One with the Author: Mr. Excuses!
By Yuri Diogenes

I have worked for more than 20 years in the IT industry, and one individual in particular sticks out in my mind. To protect this person's identity, I am going to nickname him: Mr. Excuses. I had been assigned to mentor Mr. Excuses, who was aiming to earn a higher position in the team, but in order to accomplish that he needed to learn new things. As part of this learning curve, the department had assigned for him to ramp up in some technologies. After the pre-established time that was given to him to study had passed, I felt it was time to put him in the field and see if he was ready to utilize his studies. But when I approached him with this hands-on plan, he explained he had not been able to learn the new technologies because his hands were tied with old projects, which didn't afford him time to study.

As a result, we decided to remove him from any legacy project and instead give him more time to study. We agreed on an extended timeframe (an additional 15 days), and he committed to ramping up on the new technologies. After the 15-day time period passed, I visited with him and asked if he was ready to put his knowledge into practice. Once again, he said he was not ready. But this time he blamed the lab, claiming that the computers he had to utilize in order to complete the lab didn't have enough power. In other words, he couldn't learn the new material because the machines were too slow. I made an executive decision to provide a third chance, assigning better machines to him and giving him an additional 10 days to close his learning curve. Five days after this checkpoint, he came to me and said that he was feeling too much pressure from us for him to learn, and this was affecting his health. He then proceeded to take time away from the office to deal with his health issues.

This may seem to have nothing to do with our weight-loss goal discussion, but the correlation still exists. Mr. Excuses walked through the front door of this project with the mindset of failure. We provided him with ample resources and created a precise action plan to guide him towards accomplishing his goal, but he consistently reverted to spending time and energy on the can NOT's as opposed to focusing on the CAN's and WILL's. In essence, he paved the way to failure before he ever took his first steps.

As you can see from the *One on One* anecdote you just read, spending too much mental and emotional energy on the wrong things does not allow enough energy for the action needed to progress and grow. If you constantly battle with yourself or consistently point the finger of blame in someone else's direction, you never gain introspection and never achieve forward movement towards your goals. Basically, Mr. Excuses should have allowed himself a little failure, admitted the reasons behind it, learned from the experience, and charged ahead into trying again. So remember: don't make excuses, as the only one who will be affected by those excuses is you.

There is a flipside to the "No Excuses" rule: the negative reaction of others and ultimate sabotage that others try in order to draw you into their world of making excuses to avoid success.[3] Ultimately, it is impossible to please everyone; therefore you must begin your pathway to personal change aware of this fact. While some people will applaud you in the beginning, these very same people might ignore you after they realize that you are not giving up and you are actually better than you were when you started this journey of growth. Realize that you don't have control over other people's perceptions and thoughts, so you should not let others' behavior affect your journey.

Finding the Winning Balance

Have you ever stepped out of a movie theater after being mentally glued to the big screen in the vast, dark auditorium, only to find yourself shocked that the sun is shining, that the afternoon is still lingering? You were so enthralled, so entertained, so uninterrupted in the reverie of the theater's atmosphere that you forgot what time of day it was.

We are often guilty of treating the road towards our accomplishments in this same manner. Whether we are working towards a job promotion, a college degree, a certification exam, an athletic competition, or a personal relationship, we tend to dive head first into the waters of our goal and not come up for air until the journey is completed

---

3   See a classic example of that here http://www.nydailynews. com/life-style/health/mom-3-called-bully-excuse-fitness-photo-article-1.1487278

and the goal is hopefully achieved. Unfortunately, this tends to lead to an absence of our presence in other meaningful areas of our lives. For example, a nursing student has two more years to complete her degree. During those two years, she attends classes and clinicals, lives in the library with her head buried in her books, chugs gallons of coffee, fends off sleep as much as possible, feeds the cats when necessary, feeds herself when the stomach is louder than the cats' hungry mews, and shuns friends, gym, and sun all in the name of becoming a nurse. And after two years, she wakes up one morning to find 40 pounds attached to her thighs. Dedication, drive, determination are all important key words thrown around when discussing how to attain a goal, but these three "D's" of success should not divorce one from attaining success in multiple areas of life and thus creating balance, or a "feng shui," for the interior of one's mind.

If you have ever attended a graduation speech or listened to a motivational speaker at a business conference or listened to a pep talk from a coach, then you have probably heard that you must go "all in" towards your goal. Often times, the message shouts out there is only one path to the end zone, and you have to travel that path until you plant your feet firmly past the goal line, which takes the "no excuses" mantra discussed earlier and blows it out of proportion. However, it is important to take a step back and understand that you exist in the center of something much bigger in this world.

As you can see in Figure 1-5 to the right, a personal universe made up of multiple entities surrounds you, and an existential

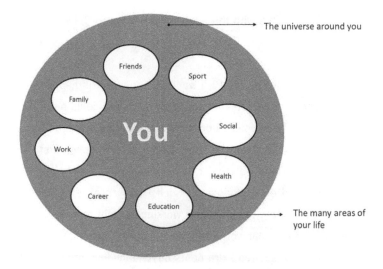

Figure 1-5: You are in the center

universe threads itself through all of that. This means that there are many areas of your life that can be controlled and many more areas of your life that cannot be personally controlled or reined in. This often leads us to having many desires or dreams. We "wish" we could affect this portion of our lives. We "wish" we could change this other portion of the world in which we live. But the difference between a desire or dream and a goal— especially a SMART goal--is that the former simply requires thought and no action and the latter requires a specific blueprint or plan of action in order to execute the changes necessary to achieve the goal.

But one must be aware that when the execution of that plan is done at the expense of many or all of the entities surrounding you, as Figure 1-5 displays, that balance is lost.

One on One with the Author: The Wakeup Call!
By Yuri Diogenes

Throughout 2009 and 2010, I went all in to make "it" happen in my career. I was determined to be the best I could be at work, and get that coveted promotion. During that same time frame, I also received the opportunity to co-write my first book to be released in the U.S. This was to be a technical book focused on a product in which I was an expert. The book required me to moonlight, working at night to write it; however, my regular work schedule did not accommodate for this, as it too required extra hours beyond the light of day in order to exceed expectations of associates higher up in the company and later lead me to that desired promotion.

As a result, I worked about 14 hours a day—from Monday to Friday—and an additional eight hours during the weekend. It was brutal! Since I had tunnel vision, with only the book deal and the career promotion in my sights, I could not see signs of things falling apart around me. I had resorted to relying on junk food as my sole source of energy, but I could not see my progressive weight gain. I could not see that I did not have (and did not make) the time to play with my kids. And I couldn't see that my private thoughts and my words in conversations encompassed only work-related matters. Looking back, I feel truly lucky to this day that I have an amazing wife who understood all reasons behind my absence and supported me as well as children who loved me unconditionally and were patient while awaiting my time and attention. My body, on the other hand, could not support the abuse and my metabolism, health, and weight all lost the weary battle and eventually gave up.

As a result, I started to feel more tired more often, though ironically I couldn't really sleep very well. Additionally, in the rare moments of playing with my youngest daughter, I could no longer run because I was unable to rapidly move a 280-pound body (with 36% body fat attached to it) without feeling intense, shooting pain in my knees. When I finally visited the doctor, my lab results were terrible: cholesterol levels had skyrocketed, and an ultrasound detected an unhealthy layer of fat around my liver. My doctor sternly told me, "You must lose weight, or you are bound to have bigger, deadlier problems."

Amidst all of this, I earned the promotion, and I published not just one but four books in 2010. So…Hell yeah! I made it happen, right? But at what expense?

That is the ultimate question. The price was just too high, and that hubris and accomplished feeling with those material achievements dissipated quickly like smoke trails on a windy day when I finally looked around and took stock in the damage left behind my work tornado. The debris slammed a reality check deep within my gut. If I wanted to truly enjoy my life, I needed to switch gears fast and make a remarkable change in my life.

When we tip the scales of our existence, like the scenario presented in the *One on One with the Author*, and the dust settles from the hard work we've put into achieving our goal at all cost, then that lack of balance reveals a void and emptiness, almost like drawing back the curtains and expecting bright blue skies outside of your window only to find complete darkness, similar to the movie theater scene that opened this chapter. Basically, the effort you pour into a solitary area of your life, at the expense of neglecting all other areas, creates an unbalanced and unhealthy environment that can create a domino effect of repercussions. Just look at Figure 1-6 below.

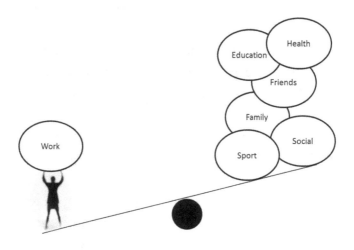

Figure 1-6: Giving 100% in one area only
will create an unsustainable balance in your life

In Figure 1-6, this person's focus is obviously only on work; he holds the responsibilities and tasks of his career like Atlas carrying the world on his shoulders; he is consequently immobilized and left with no hands to carry any other areas of his life. It looks out of balance to the naked eye when it is put into a simple pictorial; yet, it is tough to see when you are in the thick of your own moment, scrambling to achieve success at all costs. By taking a moment to examine the entire picture and give proper prioritization levels to each element as well as purposefully weighing out the cause-and-effect of pushing one area of your life over and above other areas of your life, you can maneuver more effectively towards your goals—without reaching the finish line and finding only empty air greeting you.

Flexible Winning

Let's stick with this race analogy as we move into a discussion about flexibility. Imagine you are running a 5K with a few friends on a beautiful Saturday morning, supporting a local charity. You have approximately three miles of side roads to run through hilly country. The gun goes off, people begin to trot en masse, and the wind whips through your hair as you gain speed. If you have ever run in a crowd—or for that matter, ever walked along a crowded sidewalk or even driven in rush-hour traffic madness—then you know that you cannot just continue

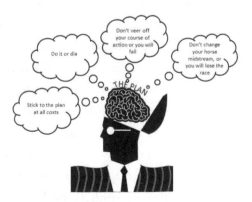

Figure 1-7: Main considerations regarding your plan of action

moving forward at your set pace and on your set straightaway path with zero mindfulness of others around you. Eventually, you will bump into someone. Instead, as you run this 5K race, you switch gears, slow your gait, shuffle your Nike-clad feet, hunker down, move to one side, move to another side, pick up speed, shorten steps, lengthen strides . . . all in accordance with the traffic that surrounds you. This is called "flexibility," a necessary component to reaching the end of any task at hand—not just ones immersed in crowded public sectors—and in a successful manner. We spoke earlier of the need to "plan" to win. Sometimes, people equate "plan" with "rigidity."

Admittedly, earlier in this chapter we introduced the "No Excuses" rule, which would seem to hint at a lack of flexibility. But don't get caught up in the locked-up approach seen above in Figure 1-7, which can actually backfire, causing a person to end up in a whirlpool of problems that they cannot escape because they keep doing what is not working. Instead, take advantage of those benchmark measurements you set up in your timeline to evaluate your progress thus far as well as examine your approach and the elements that surround you to ensure that everything is still status quo. It is at these benchmarks that you provide yourself an opportunity to shift gears, change the pace, choose a different strategy, incorporate help, and do a multitude of other activities that will all lead you towards your goal even though they may not have appeared in your original plan. Remember, just as a tree must bend its branches to move with the wind in order to avoid breakage and damage, you too need to allow for pliability and flexibility. In other words, be honest with yourself; if your plan is not working out for you, simply adjust. If the training program is too aggressive and you are having injuries every month, take your time to examine the cause-and-effect of the situation and change the program accordingly. If you have been used to poor eating habits for a decade and experience a slip up in your first two weeks, simply examine the cause-and-effect of the situation again and determine the pivotal moment that preceded the slip up. Then adjust accordingly. As you can see, it is much better to act upon things as they are happening, during the journey, rather than waiting until the end and throwing your hands up to say, "I can't; I fail," or stopping before you even started. Adaptability equals progress.

The Winds of Change

It seems like you have it all together now. A desire. A goal. A plan. Balance. Flexibility. Understanding. Now, all you need is action. But action means change, which can be scary. By moving in one direction or another, we inevitably will no longer be the same. It is a part of life. In nature, change occurs whether or not the animal or flower wishes for it. The wind blows, and a leaf falls off the tree. The sun stops shining and the flower wilts. Rain falls from the clouds above, and grass grows. A water hole dries up, and a zebra goes on the move, with a hunting lioness hot on its trails. But human beings are different. We can choose to sit in our living rooms and watch television, munching on potato chips, for as long as we wish, paying no mind to the day as it darkens or lightens. We can choose to remain in a subordinate position, meeting superior's deadlines and earning only the pay in which our contract states is our salary. We can choose to stay in the same city, continue to date the same person, enact the same bedtime ritual. Or we can challenge ourselves to move outside of the mold that our autopilot dictates and create new habits, learn new skills, earn new degrees of education, move to new places, meet new people, and essentially shed one sort of skin and allow a new sort to grow in its place.

But this is almost like choosing to jump off the side of a bridge with a bungee cord wrapped around your waist. You know you'll bounce; you know you'll experience a head rush; you know you'll scream. What you don't know for certain is where you will land or when you will stop swinging. You're told the harness is safe, the cord strong and the bridge stable. But again, you really don't know these things without a shadow of a doubt. So an element of trust is a huge part of a willingness and earnestness to jump off that proverbial bridge in your own life. You have to trust the process, the information provided, your ability to move through adversity with success, and the outcome in the end being better than the spot in which you currently reside. Changing your body, changing your skill set, changing your mental and emotional being to adhere to the process of reaching an athletic or fitness goal—as this book will demonstrate—are all rewards for accepting the challenge. It is just a matter of determining what will originate that little push that makes you move one foot and then the other off the bridge of what you were so that you can fly into the air of what you will be.

Go ahead. Jump . . . into the rest of this book and into the path of reaching your goal.

Chapter 2

BUILDING THE BEST YOU...
BRICK BY BRICK

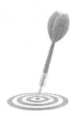

Introduction

Would you begin building a house without surveying the land upon which the foundation will be laid? Without driving through the neighborhood to witness neighbors and activity? Without examining the neighborhood drainage system? Without testing out the commute from your possible new-house location to your work? Without checking with the city zoning department for laws and regulations? Without drawing a blueprint to determine where the master bedroom will be located versus the kitchen and the subsequent plumbing lines? You get the point we are making here. Building a proper, sturdy, long-lasting house requires planning, thought, care. So, why don't we use the same approach when building ourselves?

We seem to take for granted that how we are is how we are, meaning that we see ourselves as ruled by our circumstances rather than the other way around…that our circumstances are ruled by us.

This chapter will take us through an overview of how to build our best "house" in which we will live, grow, change, progress, and nurture our livelihoods.

The Blueprint:
- Step on the sturdy parts first: Starting with right
- Checking for cracks: Moving into wrong
- Spread the mortar and fix the bricks: Putting an action plan into…action
- Maintain to sustain
- Living in your own house

Step on the Sturdy Parts First: Starting with Right
We often think that in order to solve a problem, we need to start with the problem. Returning to the house analogy that began our chapter, let us think about this in terms of discovering issues with a freshly laid foundation for a new house that sits upon shifting land. If you think this concrete slab is drying unevenly as a result, are you going to first step on the wet spots and risk getting your Nikes stuck? Or are you going to find the dry spots first and then, once you have solid footing, search for the wet spots so you can mark them from a distance and point their locations out to the builder? I would say the latter approach would be the most efficient.

One on One with the Author: It's All Inner Ear
by Jodi Leigh Miller

I once had a training client who began to experience nausea and dizziness whenever I had her perform lunges. It did not matter if she was lunging indoors—stationary style—with the Smith Machine or lunging outdoors in a traveling fashion with the dumbbells. It did not matter if the air was cool and breezy or hot and sticky. It did not matter if she had just eaten before arriving at the gym or had gone hours without food. The nausea and dizziness, accompanied by a blurred vision and kaleidoscope of stars forming behind her eyelids, made their appearance every time she lunged. I drove myself batty trying to wrack my brain in an attempt to determine the root cause of the problem.

After I had ruled out multiple sources of what she may have been doing that would CAUSE the nausea, I decided to try a different approach. I began to ask her if she experienced the nausea after leg extensions, where she was simply sitting in a chair and extending her legs at the knees. No matter how heavy the weight, the nausea and dizziness did not exist. Same thing with lying leg curls and seated leg curls. Same thing with step ups that only required her to step onto a shin-high, short box. Same thing with her warm up on the treadmill. Same thing with the majority of other exercises in her upper body workouts on other days. After listening to all of the things that we did in the gym that did *not* cause the nausea and dizzy spells, I realized that there was a common theme in the movements that preceded the nausea versus movements that did not elicit the uncomfortable state. I then asked a pivotal question: "Do you by chance have an ear infection?" She did not think she did, but she had been dealing with a small head cold for the past couple of weeks. I convinced her to go the doctor, and sure enough...she had an ear infection and needed medication. What caused the dizzy spells, sight of stars, and nausea? An absence of equilibrium due to an inner ear infection. Once the medication cleared up the infection, my client was able to lunge again without any side effects.

If I had continued to mull over the nausea and the lunges and run in circles with determining the connection between the two without ever stepping outside of those thought boundaries, my client may have either decided to quit training legs or even ended up with a severe ear infection that worsened with time and required surgery or stronger medication. But instead, I focused on moments in the workout that the nausea did not accompany. Basically, I flipped the switch on my approach to problem solving, and by focusing on what was working as opposed to what was *not* working, I helped to determine the root cause of the issue at hand and thereby led my client to a viable solution.

Checking for Cracks: Moving Into Wrong

Please do not misunderstand. In order to solve a problem, one definitely has to examine what is wrong. It just does not have to be the first step. And that is quite alright because one of the most difficult exercises that someone can do is to admit what is wrong in his or her life. Sometimes, it is easier to solve a tough question on a test when you have given yourself an opportunity to answer an easy question, and that is what this schema of examining "right" before moving into "wrong" can do for you. This approach opens up a willingness to admit to vulnerability that in turn allows a person to be honest with him or herself and thus begin laying a more balanced and stable foundation.

One on One with the Author: Why did this Happen?
By Yuri Diogenes

I distinctly remember participating in a pivotal webcast delivered by Laura Steward Atchison. She had authored the book, *What Would a Wise Woman Do? Questions to Ask Along the Way*, and her main directive for the webcast was, "ask yourself, 'why?'". And so I did. The discovery I made was astounding. I began to dig into everything I had been doing in recent years . . . even subconscious events. I traveled back in time to the point when I was 280 pounds, and I asked myself questions like: "Why did I gain so much weight?" and "Why did I do that if I was an athlete when I was teenager?" Why...why...why? As I started to track the "why" of everything, I began to learn about myself more and began to open doors to the reasons that were behind each mistake that I made along the way.

While Laura's presentation at the time was focused more on "why you will DO something," the same rationale can be used to track down the "why you DID something." We all know the old adage, "learn from your past" in order to avoid the same mistakes in your future. In my case, I was able to identify that I gained that much weight because I was in an unbalanced mode. I placed too much focus and effort into my career, and my body became merely an instrument, a vessel that carried me from one task to another while my brain did all the work. I only fed my body when I was hungry and grabbed what was most efficient and in the closest vicinity. Health? What was that? In all honesty, my health did not enter the scope of my vision when my career goals shrouded everything.

And so I kept asking myself that question of "why." Upon examining the past events, I realized way back in 2003—when I first moved to the United States alone since I could not yet bring my family—I was forced to live alone for the first time. This worked well for my laser focus upon my job, but I didn't know how to cook for myself. As a result, reliance upon fast food joints became a way of life for me. That loneliness and time away from my loved ones precipitated depression in me, and in order to fill that void, to fill a different kind of appetite, I ate...and ate...and ate.

Arriving at a clear awareness of my eating patterns and their direct connection to my mental and emotional state at the time as well as openly admitting the reasons behind the start of my downfall allowed me to mitigate this behavior in the future. Again, the tough question of "why did I do that" allowed me to make a first move in changing my behavior and working towards a better future.

This exercise of identifying what is "wrong" will enable you to establish a baseline of your most important, core areas in life. (You may refer back to Chapter 1 to help you determine these.) Once you establish this baseline, you may then identify the areas that are lower than the acceptable bar in your personal quality of life. You will see that some areas carry more pressure, stress, and/or time, which will then lead you into examining how the prioritization of this area will impact other core areas of your life.

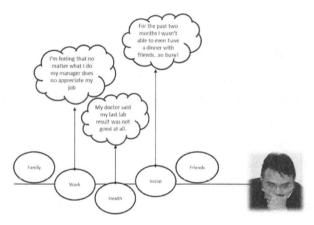

Figure 2-1: Concerns and priorities

The example shown in Figure 2-1 is one classical case of collateral damage; in other words, this man might be compromising both his health and his quality of social life because he is feeling miserable at work, where he is exerting extra effort to show his value (which sometimes includes working extra hours) and is thus unable to maintain a social life. This means that once he fixes his main issue (over-extending himself at work in a negative environment), he can then begin to mend his health issues and his social life.

Take Actions to Fix the Problem

Of course, identifying the problem is a key problem solving skill, but if you do not then determine actions to take to resolve the problem and then actually put those actions into practice, your problem will still remain...only now it is identified. Many times people carry the thought process, "It is what it is." In other words, they accept the problem lying down and resolve themselves to suffering within the quagmire. The problem will never be resolved for these people. Instead, understand that the first step to fixing a problem is to simply believe you are capable of overcoming your obstacles. Think about it. If you cannot believe in your own capabilities, change will never occur and you will forever ride the hamster wheel of distress and failure.

On that note, let us take a practice run by returning to Figure 2-1 and working to resolve the three unbalanced areas, assuming we have all the information we need to understand the overall scenario.

Health

We will tackle the health bucket from Figure 2-1 first. Ultimately, when you don't feel good—when your body is not responding properly—it affects all other areas of your life and prohibits you from mobility, timeliness, and effectiveness in all other aspects of your life. Many people take a reactionary route when it comes to their health, waiting until they experience symptoms or they receive negative news, prompting a health scare. Others may procrastinate and postpone starting healthy habits, waiting for Monday to arrive or the start of the New Year to pop up in their calendars. Still others will wait for a specific event in their lives, thus seeing health as an option rather than a necessity. The fact of the matter is, most of these people who wait to take care of themselves will not succeed because consistency and habit are lacking. Instead, if we look at health as one of our core areas—a bucket that must be filled as often as we fill a dog's water bowl—then we prolong our lives and our livelihood.

The man in Figure 2-1 is one such example of a reactionary individual who waited for negative lab results from his doctor. Inevitably, he will need to take immediate action in order to reverse the damage done. Below are three parts of the proverbial health pie:

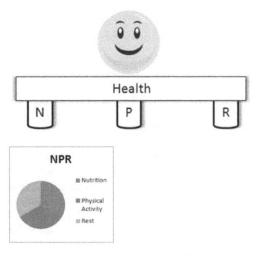

Figure 2-2: NPR as pillars for your health

Applying these principles of balancing the NPR to immediately see changes in your health is the core foundation to living better as exhibited in Figure 2-2.

- **Nutrition**: Having a balanced diet[4]
- **Physical Activity**: Exercising daily[5]
- **Rest**: Sleeping between seven to eight hours a day[6]

Just remember: if you don't make time to have a balanced NPR, you will inevitably be forced to find the time and money to treat yourself once your health is fully compromised and/or diminishes.[7]

Work

Moving into the second bucket, work, which is the place where you spend the majority of your day, which means whatever emotional stage exists at work, this is the same emotional state that will bleed into all other areas of your life. Continuing with the man in Figure 2-1, you can see he has begun a slippery slope of depression due to feeling unworthy

---

4   Read chapter 3 for more information about nutrition.

5   Exercise is fundamental part of be happier with yourself. A good read around this subject can be found it here http://www.businessinsider.com/the-single-most-proven-way-to-get-smarter-and-happier-2014-1

6   A good study about that can be found it here http://www.jsonline.com/news/health/studies-say-7-8-hours-of-sleep-is-needed-for-best-health-b9936714z1-212691521.html

7   Before beginning any exercise routine, taking any supplements, or adopting any nutrition plan, make sure that you have professional guidance and/or doctor approval.

and expendable by a boss who utilizes negative reinforcement and constant criticism in the workplace. This will be a very difficult situation for the man to overcome, but it can be done if he is dedicated to finding the root cause of the problem and creating a solution. Individuals in situations like the man in Figure 2-1 may think they must work harder and longer to achieve the results their demanding bosses require, but that is not the case. Working smarter, determining where you can make the most impact, and focusing on what you can control in your situation rather than what you cannot control—after communicating openly with management—will create a more positive and efficient work atmosphere.

There is another way to look at the issue that the man in Figure 2-1 is facing. When attempting to determine the root cause of the problem, he might discover there actually isn't a problem. Misinterpretation or self-criticism may actually be to blame. So asking a question like, *"Are you sure that your manager does not appreciate your job, or are you the one constantly seeking acceptance?"* may be helpful. It just might be this man is experiencing a lack of confidence, is questioning his own abilities, or is afraid to take risks and share ideas for fear of others' reactions. Sometimes, looking inward rather than outward can solve a great deal of stressors in the workplace and dissipate clouds of pressure and negativity. Just like waiting to take care of your health leads to a storm of issues in the long run, not fully jumping into your work with a renewed fire and a positive energy can also hold you back career-wise.

One on One with the Author:
Jump into the Fire to Spark Your Success
By Jodi Miller

Before making a career switch into personal training, I used to work for a non-profit, education reform organization. And even before that, I had been a teacher for years as well as served in management in the corporate sector. Everywhere I went, performance reviews were a yearly or bi-yearly ordeal. Yes. I said, "ordeal." My heart would race, my palms would sweat, my jaw would clench when it came time to be observed, reviewed, and dissected as a teacher or as a worker. A self-proclaimed perfectionist, I wanted the highest ratings on my reviews. I had been accustomed to earning "exceed expectations" ratings in most roles of my career history. Upon moving into the non-profit sector, I landed in a pool of overachievers just like myself, and what had exceeded expectations in my previous lines of work now netted only "meets expectations" ratings. My drive subsequently detoured and slightly stalled. I only saw "average" blinking like a neon light in Times Square when I read through my performance review, and I criticized my own performance and felt immobilized when I tried to tackle new tasks after the performance review period.

Luckily, I worked with two amazing and talented women, and once I finished licking my torn-ego wounds, I began to open my eyes and examine their performances rather than negatively focusing on my downfalls. It always helps to look one level above you or at the strongest people beside you in your workplace and study their best practices and their performance output in order to cull their positive energy (or "mojo," if you will) into your workspace. I saw them targeting the specific areas in their performance review reports and setting up plans of action to bump themselves into the next highest category of success.

I then set out to do the same for myself.

One performance area of improvement I needed to focus on was taking risks and putting my ideas on the table—with specific rationale behind those ideas. My manager could tell that while I had good ideas, I was hesitant in sharing them or didn't really fight for what I believed in. I sometimes tentatively suggested a route to take and then backed off at the first note of opposition from her. She wanted me to jump into the fire, but with a strategy in hand of how to fan those flames. So I set forth working on this very element of my performance: not backing down when I truly believed in a particular idea of mine—even if it opposed hers. By the next performance review, I netted an "exceed expectations" rating in this realm and had proven myself to be a go-getter who was willing to take strategic risks for the greater good of our educational efforts.

The moral? Don't back down or shy away from improvement. Look around you to find those who walk confidently into the workforce battle, who fan the flames of their desires to improve and achieve, and then use those sparks to create your own fires of success and positive energy in your work environment. When you do this, that very same energy will transfer into the other core areas of your life.

Ultimately, an honest self-assessment of your work environment, the expectations and responsibilities you face at work and your ultimate career goals is an imperative task to undertake. You can do this by asking yourself the following questions:

- Am I happy with the work I do, or am I just working because of the money?
- Do I wake up every day looking forward to go to work and do my job, or do I dread making the trek to work and hit the snooze button several times each morning in avoidance of starting my day?
- Does time fly at work because I am enjoying my tasks, or do I scrutinize each tick of the clock?

If your answers are predominantly in the negative for these questions, then it is highly likely you are not happy in your job. Thus, some soul-searching, re-examination of career goals, and new job hunting must take place, or the current negative environment will bleed into all other areas of your life, including your health.

Social

Social time is truly a relative term and can be defined as time spent with family and/or friends at restaurants, home-gatherings, golfing outings, shopping excursions or as time spent doing solitary hobbies such as reading, painting, watching movies, or hiking. Either way, everyone needs downtime spent away from work and necessary, daily tasks. No matter the event or activity, relaxing, reflecting, laughing, sharing, and conversing all aid in resetting one's mind and body and recharging a person for the next busy day or event in his or her life. When one's social existence becomes neglected, it creates a domino effect that triggers depression, anxiety, rise in cortisol levels due to little or no stress relief, and a loss of focus in one's goals for the workplace and health arena. The dominoes topple further because the more one feels unsuccessful in the workplace and the more one complains of headaches, loss of appetite, weight gain, and sluggishness, the less likely that person is to spend time with friends and family as well as on their own hobbies that actually alleviate these aforementioned ailments.

When examining all three categories of this man's life in Figure 2-1—work, health, and social habits—we can see that all three are interconnected. It is only through self-reflection that this man will be able to determine the root cause of his problems and be able to brainstorm solutions. If the ultimate issue in this man's life is work related, then fixing that area will positively affect his health and his social space. Rather than spinning his wheels by simply affixing a bandage on the wounded areas of his life, he can create change by going right to the source of the issue and resolving that piece of the puzzle. So for yourself, set aside quality time to examine your core areas, determine what is out of balance, and hunt down the root cause of the imbalance so you can move into the next step of actively creating solutions.

Maintaining a Balanced State

Once you have equalized all areas of your life, it would seem that you can settle into your life like a comfortable couch and ride a sleepy wave of status quo. But just as we have to constantly fill our cars with gas, check the tires for air, change the oil, and bring all liquids to their proper levels in general maintenance fashion, we must do the same for our core areas in our lives. This is actually *not* the time to sit back and relax but instead the time to hunker down and work even harder to start exceeding in each of those core areas. Now, many people believe that they can only master one area in their lives and must let the rest falter. This may be true for some, but you can choose to prioritize your core areas and determine into which one you will place 100% effort versus which ones you will place 90% or even 75% effort versus which ones you will place little to no effort since they will automatically reap the benefits simply by you being at the top of your game in the other core areas. Let's return back to the man in Figure 2-1. If he determines that work is the most important core area in his life and he has figured out that this particular job is no longer taking him in the direction of his goals, he could decide to fix the root cause of his problem by putting 100% effort into revamping his resume and starting a job search. He may put 80% of his effort into improving his health by purchasing a gym membership, hiring a personal trainer, and investing in a nicotine patch to stave off cigarette cravings. But he might put only 5% effort into making plans with friends. He is ultimately choosing to put his efforts into the core areas that he sees need to be fixed immediately and trusting that switching to a new job that is more aligned to his career goals may create a more productive atmosphere that allows him time in the future to spend with friends and family. He is thus taking control of his life, just as you can do with yours.

You should never interpret this as a way to say: *"I'm not going to give 100% of me for this project because I read that you should not forget the other areas of your life."* This is definitely not the point; the point is to evaluate *each scenario* and understand the *risks* that align themselves with the amount of effort you put into each task, just as we explained in the first chapter. You can sacrifice short-term comfort to have a long-term gain and this is not a negative; what is negative is to use this as your mantra and make it your standard behavior. When you put blinders on and create habits that have you successfully achieving only one solitary goal at the expense of other goals and core areas of your life, you risk crumbling the very infrastructure that surrounds you (for example, your family) and returning yourself to the domino effect that we mentioned earlier in this chapter. Remember: there are others that you must consider; it is not only about you. Thus, achieving your best also means ensuring the people you love feel the love back from the person that you are becoming in the midst of excelling.

One on One with the Author: Life Isn't Just About What You Did Do; It's Also About What You Didn't Do

By Yuri Diogenes

I distinctly remember an afternoon back in 2013 when I was playing with my youngest daughter, who was five years old at the time. My oldest daughter watched us as she sat perched on our living room sofa. She made a comment that I will never forget: "I don't have memories of you playing with me like you do with her now." The comment, so stark and so simple, floored me and left me speechless mainly because I knew what she said was true. When she was young, I used to work three shifts a day, oftentimes leaving home early in the morning, while the sky was still dark and she was still sleeping, and not return home until the sky had returned to dark and she was back to sleeping. I worked as a consultant during the day and a university professor teaching classes each weeknight, which meant I could only spend time with my daughter on the weekends.

After a moment of silence passed, I took a deep breath and explained to her why I did that. I needed to work those extensive hours in order to provide a better life for her— for my family. She stated that she understood my rationale. But after that moment passed, I continued my reflection to determine if what I did was truly necessary at the time. Did I really need that amount of money? Why did I need three shifts instead of two? I know the sacrifice was worth it from the professional, career-oriented standpoint since I didn't want to pass up the stellar opportunity of being a professor at a university, which ultimately put a gold star onto my resume and helped me to network and propel my career. But was the sacrifice worth it from a personal standpoint? Did I miss out on one aspect of my life by vigorously stepping up the ladder of success in another aspect of my life?

I could go back and forth in this dilemma, and I'm not sure there is just one right answer. Instead, we must conclude that sacrifices are inevitable and necessary. The key is you have to be aware and accepting of the fact that no matter which route you take, there will be consequences to face. Ensure that you brainstorm each route before you begin traveling down the road of achieving your goals. Create a cost-benefits analysis chart for yourself and then realize that as long as you are aware of the risk and willing to take it and face the consequences head on while also attempting to minimize the damage that such decision will cause, then you should have no wavering and no regrets. Just always keep in mind that for the loved ones around (parents, children, significant others, friends), life is not just about what you do for them but also what you didn't do with them. Your actions speak louder than your words, so be present in the moment, give them undivided attention, and express your love for them in ways that they understand. Keep an open channel of communication so they feel comfortable in letting you know they need more time or more action from you, and in turn you feel comfortable in explaining your daily rituals and how they connect to future goals. We become role models to our loved ones when we treat our sacrifices in this manner.

During this maintenance phase you have two choices: *turn on the cruise control and always keep this balance* or *take risks once in awhile that could cause an unbalanced state*. Both options will net positive results but in different respects, and it really depends on each individual and his or her ultimate goals in life. The only thing you must understand is that if you do not challenge yourself and if you do not take risks, you will stagnate in life and not grow. It is normal for your life to feel like a rollercoaster at times; ups and downs are a part of the growth process, as you can see below in Figure 2-3. Sometimes you have to step back from the microscopic view of the present moment in time, look at the big picture, and then move forward once you have reset your vision. This step back doesn't mean a regression; rather, it means that you are approaching your life by looking at different angles as part of your strategy to keep growing.

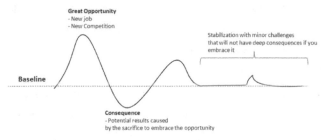

Figure 2-3: Creating a baseline

The unbalanced state will happen if you take risks to grow in certain areas of your life, but remaining aware and facing the fact that temporary sacrifices may pop up will help you to mitigate and alleviate the damage. Thus, every time that you see an opportunity to go to a better place, which could be a better position at work or preparing for a competition, you should use the "HWH" technique explained in the first chapter.

Transforming the Change to a Lifestyle

As you make changes in order to live better and build a better you, it will be normal that the first few months you will struggle to remain consistent. Change is not easy; even when you have all the right reasons to change, your old habits will still come back once in a while to disrupt you. The most classic example is dieting to lose weight. Many people will start a diet by thinking ahead to what they will eat once they achieve their goal and how they can return back to their old habits. This is a faulty mindset because the weight will slowly creep back in and these people will be back to square one. Instead, it is important to embrace the change and turn it into a lifestyle rather than a temporary fix.

There is a lifestyle-change theory floating about that if you consistently do something for 21 days, that action will become a habit. This theory has been debunked[8] by many researchers; in our personal experiences, it took way more than 21 days for either of us to make a habit a true lifestyle change. On the flip side, researchers[9] have also determined that habits are indeed malleable and flexible. So you should never assume that just because you have an old habit, you cannot get rid of it. This really is a case-by-case situation, dependent upon the habit itself,

---

8   Here an excellent article that demystify this theory http://blog. neatandsimple.com/2007/06/mythbusting_new.html

9   You can find the results of this research here http://web.mit.edu/ newsoffice/2012/understanding-how-brains-control-our-habits-1029. html

your willingness to make a change occur, and the consistent effort you place in creating a new habit.

One on One with the Author:
The First 90 Days of Change,
By Yuri Diogenes

When I decided to change my lifestyle in October, 2011, I first decided that I couldn't see this as just one solitary attempt since I had failed numerous times in the past to change my eating habits. I instead had to reverse my thinking from day one and see this as an overhaul to my lifestyle. Upon reflection, I realized that my previous attempts to lose weight were unsuccessful because I only focused upon losing the weight and watching the numbers go down on the scale. I had to change my outlook and instead see this as a way to start a new me and a new way of living.

The first week of the new nutrition and training plan was probably the worst ever: headaches, cramps, weak moments, disconnection from co-workers and family members, and cravings were all symptoms through which I had to suffer. I had made a sudden and drastic switch from a life full of junk food, freedom of caloric choices, and approximately 5,000 calories per day to a rigid plan that allowed 1,800 calories per day with specific breakdowns of 60% protein, 30% carbohydrates, and 10% fat. As the side effects reared their ugly heads during that first week, my mind had to take hold and become strong and focused on my goals. I wanted permanent change, not just a change in numbers on the scale. I wanted a new lifestyle, a new me. So I had to fight the urges, temptations, and discomforts in order to create new habits that would carry me through the rest of my life . . . a healthy life.

After 90 days on this new regimen, my weight had dropped almost 40 pounds! I had started the plan at 260 pounds and found myself staring at 223 pounds on the scale. While I knew this was not a numbers game, I also understood that I was achieving the best results I had ever had with a weight loss plan. But even better news is that in those 90 days, I essentially changed my lifestyle; I actually began to enjoy eating the foods on my plan and began to look forward to my workouts six days per week. I did not just bask in that short-term success. I continued going after the larger goal, and after seven months,[10] I became a completely different person. Those junk foods I mentioned earlier no longer swam in front of my eyes; I didn't want to "cheat" on my plan, for that would be me "cheating" on my goals. I simply wanted to continue eating and exercising in the manner that was working wonders for me.

---

10   You can see the results of seven months transformation here
https://www.youtube.com/watch?v=LYkRJDFexhM

Chapter 3
ENLIGHTENING THE MIND AND ACTIVATING THE BODY THROUGH EXERCISE AND NUTRITION

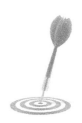

Introduction

Ask ten people how they pack a suitcase for a trip, and you will invariably get ten different answers. Some haphazardly fling clothes into the yawning mouth of a canvas bag with no rhyme or reason. Others take a calculated inventory of their closet, pull out every single possible item that *might* work for the trip, and then pack as much as possible, only removing items when the zipper threatens to break on the overstuffed suitcase. But no matter the method, the fact remains that all people packing a suitcase need to bring the same categories of essentials: clothes, shoes, identification, and money.

Training and dieting are very much like packing for a trip. There are categories of essentials that fit across the board, no matter the goal and no matter the person. But the methods used by each individual person will vary greatly. Just as not every person is flying to the same city and not every person is traveling for the same purpose, like a work conference or a honeymoon or a winter vacation, not every person wants to fit into the same size jeans and not every person wants to actually compete in an athletic event. This is why the background information presented in Chapters 1 and 2 is so important in terms of determining needs, goals, resources, and an overall plan of action. Once you capture those items, you can then commit yourself to concrete work towards those goals.

So…remember Tyler Durdan in *Fight Club*? The first rule of packing your own suitcase is there are no rules. And thus, the first rule of training and dieting (besides not calling it "die"ting) is there are no rules . . . only suggestions to observe, lessons to learn, observations to make, and results to be had.

Self-Awareness

Speaking of observations, take a moment to become aware of your body right now, in this very moment as you read this chapter. How are you breathing? What are your eyelids doing? Where are your hands? How are your legs crossed? Do you have an itch? Are other thoughts running through your mind as you simultaneously read these words? How are you reading these words (i.e., one at a time or collectively as a whole sentence or paragraph)? These questions trip you up, don't they? The moment you begin to examine your breathing is the moment you begin to breathe purposefully. The moment you determine what your hands are doing is the moment you probably stop twirling your hair or picking at a scab or tapping on the desk. This is the very same thing that occurs when we become self-aware in the gym and in the kitchen. We become purposeful. We actively make decisions rather than passively move through auto-piloted motions.

In the education world, this is termed as "metacognition," otherwise known as an awareness of why you are thinking what you are thinking. For teachers in classrooms, this is an important tool because it allows a teacher to recognize when students do not comprehend a concept and then alter his or her delivery to fit individual students' needs directly in the moment of the lesson. It definitely goes deeper than this when discussing the education sector, but if we transfer this idea into the fitness sector, we open a whole world of possibilities for enabling and empowering a person to recognize what his or her body is doing directly during exercise in the gym and to become aware of what a person is eating and why he or she is eating that food item in that very moment.

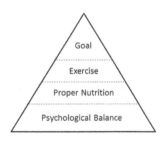

Figure 3-1: The "change pyramid"

This is the psychological aspect to effecting long-term change. If we design a hierarchy, or a "change pyramid" as displayed in Figure 3-1 above, to the most important components of designing change in one's lifestyle, the psychological aspect becomes the foundation—or heart and soul—of the matter. Often times, people make a mistake of jumping into the deep end of nutrition and training and then drown in a pool of mistakes and disappointments because they rushed into the action steps without truly examining how they feel and perceive themselves and what they are about to accomplish.

Enacting self-awareness in the following four categories essentially creates a life preserver:

- Mind
- Body
- Food
- Exercise

Mind

How much control do you have over your mind? Can you change your thoughts midstream? When you wake up late in the morning because you didn't hear your alarm, the hot water heater has broken and only cold water spouts out of the shower head, the kids are arguing with each other, you spill coffee on your white shirt, and the oatmeal boils over in the microwave, can you stop the rush of negativity entering your mind and take a deep breath while telling yourself, "It's okay; this will all be a memory in a short while"?

Control over the mind requires an awareness of one's own thought process, an ability to recognize the path in which the mind is traveling, and a concerted effort to change the direction of the thoughts should they guide us down a useless or derogatory path. Typically, what we believe is exactly what we will achieve, so if we see ourselves as having a bad day because of the morning's collective fiasco, then the drive to work will be a stressful one; you'll walk into work with your heart racing, teeth gnashing, and voice barking orders at your colleagues. You might end up complaining to your assistant about how this day got off to a rough start and as a result pull the focus off of the project's deadline for that day. A domino effect of negativity will fall into place. But if you can stop and say, "one event does not necessarily affect another event unless I allow it," then you can change your entire mindset and enable a more open and productive self to rise up for the day.

Part of the success of doing this involves visualization. By taking a step back and seeing yourself in a productive, successful manner throughout each major task of the day ahead, you set yourself up for success and actively change your mindset. For example, instead of fuming on the way to work during rush hour traffic and glaring down at the coffee stain on your white shirt, turn your focus to your afternoon presentation and seeing yourself talking to the table of co-workers and flowing through the PowerPoint with ease and no technological difficulties. Move your vision into a later point in the day where you see yourself driving to the gym, singing to one of your favorite tunes that gets you ready for your workout, and then actually lifting the weights and even blasting through a new personal record with your squats or bench press. It is highly likely you will perform each one of these tasks with exactly the fervor and success that you envision during your drive into work, AND your day at work will be more positive and more productive, thus killing two birds with one stone.

One on One with the Author: If You Build It In Your Head, It Will Come True
by Jodi Leigh Miller

I began competing in physique competitions during a time when only two divisions existed: Fitness and Bodybuilding. I had no dance or choreography background to do well in Fitness and was not big enough in muscle size or stature for Bodybuilding at the time. But I desperately wanted to look like the women I saw in magazines like *Oxygen* and *Muscle and Fitness*. And I wanted to bring that look to the stage. At the time, the only other venue to do such an activity was The Galaxy Federation, which was an organization that combined an obstacle course round on one day with a bikini round on the second day. This was perfect for me, except for one thing: I was—and still am—petrified of heights, and the obstacle course required a 15-foot high cargo net to be climbed and a 10-foot wall to be attacked via a rope.

I originally attended a camp to learn how to scale both apparatuses, but the actual practice did nothing to assuage my fears. I literally saw myself toppling off the top of the cargo net or accidentally letting go of the rope and falling to the hard ground below. I imagined broken bones, a concussion, torn muscles, and a whole slew of horrific occurrences just from being a part of this obstacle course competition.

A friend of mine, Eric Jones, who was a high school strength and conditioning coordinator at the time and helping me with sprint and plyometrics drills in order to prepare for the competition, convinced me to change my mindset and stop imagining the bad stuff from happening. So every night during my competition prep, I would lay in bed, close my eyes, and imagine myself running the course: swift like a cheetah, elegant like a gazelle, fearless as a monkey swinging through trees in a jungle. I visualized that race from start to finish, scrambling up the cargo net, flipping to the other side, scurrying down, racing to the rope wall, pulling myself up with ease, dropping to the ground with nary a scratch, and finishing the remainder of the course without a hitch. I would visualize this scenario at least three times every night leading up to the competition.

Now, I didn't actually move like any of those animals I mentioned when it came time for the real event. I still had an utter fear of heights that to this day has not dissipated. But I did run through the obstacle course—even if it was more like a sloth—and took each of my turns at the course during each competition and never backed down no matter how much my heart pitter pattered and my fear tried to choke me. I even conquered a competition that was just two weeks after I had met my fear head on and fallen off of the cargo net from almost 15-feet in the air during practice. As you can see, giving my mind permission to view success, to see the positive, gave strength to my performance in a way that negative thought cannot. What we think, how we think...this truly does determine our future.

Body

When was the last time you looked at your body? Really looked at it? Not just glaring into the foggy mirror as you hurry out of the shower and into your towel to dry off. Not just to find the dastardly stray hairs in the most inopportune spots on your body to tweeze out. Not just a quick gander as you hop into bed and wonder why the squishy section on your belly will not disappear no matter how many crunches you do. No, none of that. Instead, really look at your body, without clothes. Examine and touch and peer and see. Study and commit to memory. The good and the not so good.

But then go one step further. Touch the areas that you wish to work upon and improve. Commit the feel of your muscle to memory. Know how your thighs, your butt, your arms, your shoulders, your stomach, your lower back all feel beneath your fingertips. Commit to memory the softness that may be in the way of revealing that muscle. It is in this manner you will know your starting point and can actively measure your progress. You will have a direct memory—based upon touch and sight—of your body when you perform in the gym or on the track or on a treadmill.

Food

How often do you pop a Jolly Rancher or peppermint candy into your mouth at a work meeting or say yes to a frappe sample at the coffee shop or accept a bite of a cookie that a friend offers to you at a gathering? Do you know how long it has been since your last meal? Do you ever skip breakfast because you are in a hurry or are not hungry? Have you ever chewed down on an entire bag of chips in zombie fashion, only awakening when your greasy fingers hit the rock bottom of salty crumbs and slippery foil? Do you ever open the refrigerator and blankly stare at the array of chilled contents only to grab a package of lunchmeat and munch mindlessly? Do you know why you didn't say no to that piece of cake after dinner? Or better yet, do you know why you *did* say no to that piece of cake after dinner?

Try this for one week: write down on paper or type into your smartphone every single item that goes into your mouth, including food, gum, and liquids. This is called journaling. If you can do it in the moment as much as possible, you are advised to include the activity and emotion(s) surrounding the time period in which you have eaten or drunk something. Take inventory at the end of the week to see what and when you are actually eating and drinking. If we do not record our actions and actively draw our own attention to them, we create a distorted, biased, selective, or forgetful view of what we did. Without a tangible recording of our actions, we also cannot observe trends over a period of time; we cannot determine a correlation between what we are doing, what we are feeling, and what we are eating or drinking. Once you have history truthfully recorded, you can discern the patterns of behavior, see clearly what needs to change as opposed to what needs to stay the same, and subsequently work on a plan of action.

Exercise

We are funny-looking creatures when we exercise. Our grunts, grimaces, groans, and goings-on do not always paint a beautiful picture. Our limbs flail about, our faces contort, our armpits sweat. We can look around at others and giggle at the sights we see as people push through their exercises. But can we look at ourselves and know what our bodies are doing in the moment? Do you know if your knees buckle in as you squat? Do you know that your elbows flare out inadvertently when you do bench dips for your triceps? Do you know that you heavily shift to one hip when you run? Do you realize that your traps tense up when you try to work on shoulders? How would you know these things? Well, there are a few different tools you can use.

1. *Stimulation via Touch:* If you have a workout partner or trainer, this is an excellent method for getting the brain to fire off neurons to the precise site being worked. Simply have your partner or trainer take their index and middle fingers and place the tips of them directly on the muscle that should feel the tension from the exercise. For example, if you are training biceps and doing alternating dumbbell curls, have your partner or trainer place their fingertips directly on the peak of the bicep. Your attention is now guided towards the bicep peak and away from the ache in your back, the itch on your ankle, the tightness in your shoulders.

2. *Stimulation via Vision:* The mirrors in the gym are not there for primping purposes, even though there are always a few peacocks in the gym who use them

for just that reason. They are actually there so you can watch your form and observe the movements from your body as you perform the exercise. For example, if you are doing a seated overhead dumbbell press, you can use the mirror to determine if your elbows are at a 90-degree angle, if your forearms are perpendicular to the floor, and if your chest is elevated and not dropped when you are in the starting position of the exercise. You can continue to watch to see if your traps take over as you press the dumbbells up and over your head. Then you can fix the issues in real time. One other tool to use is video. Most people these days have an excellent camera on their phones. Have your workout partner or trainer take a video of you performing the exercise at hand. Watch it together afterwards and evaluate it, pointing out the positives and noting the movements to fix. Then you go into your second set with a visual awareness of what to improve or correct.

3. *Stimulation via Flexing:* If you can flex a muscle when you are not holding weight, then you are more than likely going to be able to flex the muscle when performing a weight-related exercise. Practice one muscle at a time, posing and pumping much like a bodybuilder, in order to understand and feel the muscle doing the work. Commit that feeling to memory and then utilize that memory when you are in the gym and working that same muscle group with weight.

4. *Stimulation via Verbalization:* If you can teach it, you can learn it. Take the time to explain to someone else

what you are doing and why you are doing it while you are doing it in the gym. As you describe what your body is supposed to do and where you are supposed to feel it, your mind will automatically travel to those very actions and those very spots on the body. It will bring awareness that will allow you to correct as you go. Ideally, you would do this during warm up or lighter sets to avoid injury, but the self-awareness and subsequent correction will arise in enough time for you to be successful in your heavier lifts.

You are now set to begin work on the foundation of your own change pyramid. Be sure to read the last portion of this chapter for specific technology tools that aid these aspects of creating and maintaining yourself awareness, including community forums, food journals, and exercise logs.

Nutrition and Training

Before we do delve into those specific tools, we must first tackle the meat of your change pyramid: nutrition and training. Successfully creating self-awareness in the fitness and health aspect is almost a Catch 22 scenario. You have to be aware of what you are doing in order to know how to change it. But you have to learn the basics of nutrition and training in order to fully build your self-awareness. This section of the chapter will provide you with bare essentials of knowledge. There are entire courses, books, and degrees that focus on each of these two areas. In addition, there are many methods people may use to get in shape. Some people rely upon the "Do It Yourself"

(DIY) approach, in which they use minimum guidance to achieve a goal. This may include reading articles, watching videos, and applying learned principles to their daily activities without ever hiring a trained professional. But for most people, we highly recommend that you seek professional assistance in the beginning, primarily from a doctor and a certified trainer. As discussed in the previous chapter, it is important to know your current physical and health condition, which involves getting your blood work done. This also builds an assessment and understanding of your body to see which physical activities you can perform and where you lag in joint and stability performance. Although there are commonly used programs and so-called standard diets, each person will react differently for each program, thus creating varying results that may or may not match with your original fitness or performance goals.

Therefore, our goal as authors is not to teach you— the reader—*how* to eat or *how* to train but instead to bring awareness about best practices that currently exist and to provide tools and resources that will get you on track as well as keep you there while you work towards your health, fitness, and competitive goals. This section will be designed to provide basic definitions and couple them with specific tools and resources to help you gain knowledge that is designed specifically for your unique goals.

Nutrition

Balance is key when it comes to the types of foods we choose for our daily diet (these types of foods are also known as macronutrients). But assessing your starting point with a professional, determining your unique goals, and discussing with that professional the proper route to take toward a specific competition, sport, or end result of weight loss or muscle gain are just as important as that term "balance." Bodybuilders may need more protein than marathon runners, and mixed martial arts (MMA) fighters might need more carbohydrates than golfers. Someone who is 6'2" and 181 pounds will have a different macronutrient structure than someone who is 5'2" and 160 pounds. Keep this in mind as you read through the terms listed below; then, peruse the tools and resources provided here and take advantage of them as you need in order to reach your goals.

What is Your Healthy Weight?

Unfortunately, we cannot answer this question decisively for you. At one point, BMI (Body Mass Index) was a term cemented in certainty. It is determined by the following steps:

1. Multiply your weight in pounds by 0.45
2. Multiply your height in inches by 0.025
3. Divide the number from step 1 by the number in step 2.
4. Or you can visit http://www.nhlbi.nih.gov/health/ educational/lose_wt/BMI/bmicalc.htm to enter in your information and examine the chart provided.

The caution nowadays against using BMI as more than a subordinate tool is grounded in the fact that BMI does not take into account one's body composition (comprised of the location and amount of body fat), lean muscle tissue, and overall genetics. A 4'11" professional female bodybuilder who is 7% body fat and weighs 120 pounds carries a very different BMI than a 4'11" amateur female golfer who is 21% body fat and weighs 118 pounds. Be sure the professional you choose to help you attain your goals does not rely solely on BMI when determining your caloric intake.

Calorie

This is a unit of energy, originating from three groups of nutrients (protein, carbohydrates, fats). Once these nutrients—found in the foods you eat—are digested, they then convert to glucose (or blood sugar) once they hit the bloodstream. Your body needs calories every day in order to sustain living. Determining just how many calories you need is dependent upon your body's make up (height, weight, age) as well as your activity level throughout the day.[11] The more you move, the more calories you need. The more muscle you have, the more calories you need. So beware of fad diets or professionals that try to drastically restrict calories. If you go too low in your calories, your body could fight against you and begin storing those calories in order to protect itself, making fat loss almost impossible. In addition, not all calories are equal in how they react to your particular

---

11 You can determine your BMR (basal metabolic rate) by visiting this link: http://www.bmi-calculator.net/bmr-calculator/. You can take it a step further and calculate your BMR by the number assigned to your relevant activity level. This will inform you regarding an estimate of the number of calories you need in order to sustain yourself at that activity level per day. This is, of course, an estimate and a professional's guidance is always recommended to ensure proper caloric intake and nutrition levels are being met daily.

body's unique structure and overall needs. So also beware of any fad diets or professionals that preach a basic "calorie in/calorie out" approach. For most athletes, whether you are preparing for a triathlon, a golf tournament, a tennis match, a cross-country cycling event, a powerlifting meet, or a bodybuilding show, a more individualistic nutrient structure is needed since fat loss, muscle mass gain, endurance, and strength goals vary by sport.

Protein

The general definition of a protein is: "any of various naturally occurring extremely complex substances that consist of amino-acid residues joined by peptide bonds, contain the elements carbon, hydrogen, nitrogen, oxygen, usually sulfur, and occasionally other elements (as phosphorus or iron), and include many essential biological compounds (as enzymes, hormones, or antibodies)."[12] This long-winded definition probably will not stick in anyone's mind except those with science or nutrition degrees, so it is helpful to understand that a protein is important because it is used "to build and repair body tissues, to make enzymes, hormones, and other body chemicals; to transport nutrients; to make your muscles contract, and to regulate body processes such as water balance."[13] Additionally, proteins are divided into two major groups: complete proteins and incomplete proteins. A complete protein contains the entire chain of essential amino acids, which are the building blocks of proteins, but incomplete proteins are missing at least one of the essential amino acids. Examples of complete proteins

---

12 http://www.merriam-webster.com/dictionary/protein
13 American Dietetic Association's Complete Food and Nutrition Guide

include poultry, fish, meat, eggs. Examples of incomplete proteins include grains, nuts, beans, seeds, and corn. If you are a vegetarian or a vegan, it is important to have a professional helping you to find the correct combination of incomplete proteins in order to take in a more complete chain of essential amino acids within each meal. Finally, for every gram of protein ingested, four (4) calories are supplied.

Carbohydrates

Carbohydrates are brain food. Typically, when broken down, they provide the body with energy needed to sustain daily activities. They usually are in the form of sugars and starches or otherwise known as simple carbohydrates and complex carbohydrates. Various forms of sugar such as table, cane, and brown sugars as well as honey and agave fall into the category of simple carbohydrates. Refined sugars found in soft drinks and candies are also considered simple carbohydrates. Whether processed or refined, simple carbohydrates need to be utilized very quickly for energy, or they run the risk of turning to fat at a quicker rate than complex carbohydrates, which include foods like potatoes, sweet potatoes, corn, rice, quinoa, beans, grains, oats, pasta, pumpkin, and fall squash. Everything in the complex carbohydrate category is slower to break down to sugar in the blood stream; they provide the body with longer lasting energy. There is a final category of carbohydrates known as fibrous, which are your vegetables—green, leafy, and colorful— such as broccoli, spinach, kale, asparagus, artichokes, onions, bell peppers, Brussels sprouts, zucchini, and a multitude of other vegetables. These plant foods provide fiber that supports the immune system, assists with digestion, and lowers blood sugar and cholesterol levels. For every gram of carbohydrate digested, four (4) calories are supplied to the body.

Fats

Fats also supply energy to the body and are important for insulating the body, cushioning vital organs, and aiding in brain development. They supply nine (9) calories to the body for every gram of fat digested, which is more than double the amount than the other macronutrients and make these the densest of the macronutrients. Healthy choices of unsaturated fats include nuts (like cashews, almonds, pecans, walnuts) and nut butters, avocado, flaxseed, chia seeds, and salmon, to name several.

Both carbohydrates and fats provide energy, but different people utilize these two macronutrients in unique ways, so it is important to evaluate your body, energy levels, athletic performance in terms of endurance and strength, as well as overall mood and memory in order to determine whether your diet should be richer in carbohydrates or in fats as a main energy source. Once you tap into this, your fat loss efforts will become more efficient and quicker paced. Keeping a journal—a food diary, if you will—and consulting with a professional will help you to determine this.

This actually leads us into a discussion regarding a very popular term that has been bounced around social media: "if it fits your macros." It is often seen as the acronym, "IIFYM," and can be utilized in a variety of manners. At one end of the spectrum, a person may take the macronutrient categories at face value and literally replace a carbohydrate with any other carbohydrate and a fat with any other fat and a protein with any other protein, thus coming to the conclusion that he or she may adequately and equally replace a dinner meal consisting of 6 ounces chicken breast, 1 cup basmati rice, half of an avocado, and 1 cup of broccoli with two slices of a local dive's pizza consisting of a refined, white flour crust, mozzarella cheese, olive oil, Canadian bacon, bell peppers and onions. While both contain protein, carbohydrates, and fats, the types of each of these macronutrients actually varies. Rather than taking such a holistic approach to the IIFYM, instead investigate the actual kinds of macronutrients that work best for your body and then determine the appropriate exchanges within those categories. For example, if red potatoes work very well for you as an energy-providing carbohydrate source, chances are wild rice will also do the job. Sweet potatoes would probably work too. A corn tortilla and black beans might also suffice. All of these are carbohydrates that will be utilized in a similar fashion in the body and do not carry refined or processed sugars and are longer-lasting energy sources. Again, keeping track of your food choices in an online or paper journal (a few resources will be provided later in this chapter) as well as consulting with a professional will assist you in making the best choices for exchanges of foods so that your diet has variety and provides an array of nutrients to keep you healthy. And this provides a true method to the madness of "flexible dieting."

To Cheat or Not to Cheat

There are so many terms for foods that we feel we could look at and gain weight without ever tasting a delectable morsel.

Cupcakes, brownies, gelato, French fries, macaroni and cheese, spaghetti, queso, chips, ribs. The list goes on and on. Foods that are heavily processed and packaged. Foods that are just rich in sugars and fats. Foods that sing to us like the Sirens sing to Odysseus' men, inviting us to come a little closer and take a little bite and then another bite and another bite until the plate or bag or pan is wiped clean of any remaining crumbs. We call them "cheats," "treats," "junk foods," bad foods," "dirty foods." We think we should avoid them at all costs, and yet the more we attempt to stave off temptation, the more their sweet and salty voices capture our attention and numbingly draw us in. The thing is, these foods are not all "bad" per se. In moderation, they can provide a spark to our system and to our taste buds, allowing us a breather from the diet doldrums, reviving up our metabolism, and creating a euphoria that lasts in our memory banks.

That being said, if you are eating enough and often enough, then your cravings for those "bad" or "dirty" foods will lessen considerably. In order to keep energy levels and blood sugar levels consistent and well-maintained (i.e., not dropping suddenly or spiking heavily), one must eat more often. Just like a fire needs wood or kindle added in order to keep the flames alive, the body needs food throughout the day in order to fuel its energy tank. This can mean eating anywhere from five (5) to seven (7) meals per day, especially if you are a competitive athlete preparing for an event such as a triathlon, marathon, "tough mudder" race, an intramural team event like rugby or flag football, or a bodybuilding competition. Now, that seems like a lot of chewing in one day, right? But if you break it down into simple categories of breakfast, lunch, dinner, and snacks, with each snack occurring after each main meal, then it becomes easier to handle mentally. In all actuality, by having more meals throughout the day, a person is able to eat smaller portions at one sitting but end up with a larger caloric intake overall by the end of the day. Please refer to figure 3-2 for an example:

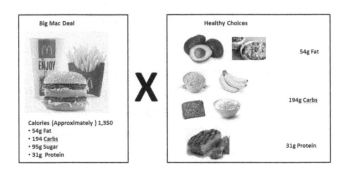

Figure 3-2: Not all calories are the same

In Figure 3-2 on the left side, we see just one meal consisting of a fast food burger, French fries, and a soft drink (presumably *not* diet, though diet soft drinks carry their own prescription of issues via artificial sweeteners). In just one sitting, a person who gobbles down this meal takes in a whopping 1,350 calories. That's over half of the suggested daily allotment of calories for many individuals. Not only that, a quarter of those calories (380 calories, to be exact) originate from refined sugars (remember, every gram of carbohydrate yields four (4) calories). The person eating this meal probably is not headed to the gym and will not utilize these calories for any particular energy-driven activity but instead find him or herself crashing in energy.

On the flip side, looking at the right side of Figure 3-2, we see just how many options of lesser-processed, more natural foods a person can choose from and actually spread out throughout the day in multiple meals. While the protein serving is approximately the same and typical of a single-sitting intake (31 grams), the fats and carbohydrates can be divided out into three to four meals throughout the day, allowing the body to better digest and process the food and appropriately utilize it for the prescribed activity of the day. Let's examine the carbohydrates a little further and compare both sides of Figure 3-2 more closely. On the left side, the carbohydrates come from refined sugars in the soft drink, as stated earlier, as well as the white bun on the burger and the French fries. In contrast on the right side, the carbohydrates come from fruit (bananas), rice, grains (whole grain bread), and oats. All 194 grams of carbohydrates included on the right side of Figure 3-1 would not be eaten in one meal but instead spread out amongst three to four meals in many cases, yielding 48 to 68 grams of carbs in one sitting rather than almost 200 grams of carbs. Essentially, less is more per meal. But the person eating the foods in the right side of Figure 3-2 also has the appetite to eat four or five more meals and thus take in more protein daily, which is important for building muscle, than the person eating the foods on the left side of Figure 3-2. This means the body is constantly being fueled throughout the day and blood sugar levels remain level rather than dipping or spiking. As a result, this person will: sleep better; deal with stress better; have better skin, nails, and hair, and will have more energy, strength and endurance for better workouts.

Now that we have a stronger handle on nutrition, we are ready to jump right into the training and exercise portion of meeting our fitness goals.

Training

"Abs are made in the kitchen." You've heard that phrase, right? In one respect, it's true. If you don't follow the aforementioned best practices of nutrition, then the fluff that sits atop of the abdominal wall will hide the muscle beneath. But if you don't work the muscle, then it will never reach its true potential of shape, size, and detail. Essentially, training and nutrition go hand in hand when creating a performance-ready or show-ready physique (even if the only show you wish to reach is the one in front of your bathroom mirror with a judge of only one—you).

Training can encompass a multitude of different types of exercises. Just like we did with the nutrition section, we will simply provide a starting point, with a few best practices and ideas that will help you get started as well as tools and resources to check out in order to reach your unique fitness and performance goals.

Cardiovascular Exercise

The first category is cardiovascular—or aerobic exercise. Aerobic exercise uses oxygen to burn carbohydrates and fats for energy. Several schools of thought exist regarding what type of cardio works best for an individual. Just like nutrition is not a one-size-fits-all entity, neither is cardio. Some people lose more weight doing "fasted" cardio[14], which is cardio performed upon waking up and prior to eating the first meal of the day. Others do not respond well to doing cardio on an empty stomach and find that they lose precious muscle and strength gains when incorporating this approach. Thus, they save the cardio work for later in the day. Some people respond well to steady-state cardio, which keeps the heart rate elevated but even keel throughout the time of performing the exercise. An example of this is walking on a treadmill at a 3.8 speed and a 3.0% incline and not changing it faster or slower for the duration of the workout. For those whom this approach does not work best, performing high intensity interval training (HIIT) will prove most beneficial and allow an individual to change variables within the exercise to bring the heart rate up and down like a roller coaster ride. This can be done by changing speed, resistance, and exercise type on an exercise apparatus. The following is a quick example of a HIIT cardio session: run on a treadmill at a 6.5 speed and no incline for 60 seconds before stepping off the treadmill to perform an explosive plyometrics move like jump squats and then pushing a weighted apparatus—like a "prowler"—as fast as you can for 40 yards and finally stepping back onto the treadmill to walk

---

14 Recent studies concluded that fasted cardio does not help burn more fat, read this article for more information http://well.blogs.nytimes.com/2011/06/27/does-exercising-on-an-empty-stomach-burn-more-fat/?_r=0; however, there are other studies mentioned by Dr. Jim Stoppani that show the opposite. Please see http://www.bodybuilding.com/fun/is-fasted-cardio-the-best-for-burning-fat.html for more information. Each person will react differently, so you must find if this method works for you.

at a speed of 3.8 with an incline set at 12% for three minutes before repeating the entire process again three more times.

Determining the ideal amount of time spent performing cardiovascular exercise as well as choosing the proper cardio equipment (like a treadmill, Elliptical trainer, recumbent bike, or Stairmaster, to name a few) or specific exercises (like plyometrics or sprinting) are ultimately dependent upon your specific needs, interests, and end goals. Your nutritional intake or plan must also be taken into consideration in order to ensure the proper caloric deficit or surplus occurs with your performance needs and goals in mind. A professional can aid you, and the weightlifting section below will delve into this further.

Weightlifting

The second category is weightlifting, which is anaerobic and does not require oxygen. It can be separated into three divisions: machines, cables, and free weights, of which all are useful to reach a well-rounded physique. Machines provide structure and stability for the body. Appearing in the form of pec deck machines, Smith machines, hack squat machines, leg press machines, and Hammer Strength pressing machines—to name a few—these all keep the body somewhat locked into a position, keeping the body from having to stabilize supporting joints in order to move the weight in a two-dimensional format. These are useful in order to create intense focus on a particular muscle and can sometimes allow for more weight to be moved because the body is held in a stationary position. On the other hand, both cables (which use a pulley system) and free weights, like dumbbells and barbells, offer a more functional approach that forces the body to stabilize itself while performing the exercise. Examples include dumbbell curls, free-bar squats, dumbbell overhead press, and seated cable rows.

It is okay if a feeling of sensory overload—much like day one of hearing a professor's lecture in a quantum physics college course—has suddenly set in after reading the above paragraph. People often step foot into a gym, look at the wide expanse of machines, cables, dumbbells, barbells, and benches, throw their hands up in confusion and frustration, and make a beeline straight for the treadmill because that is easiest to figure out. Just press "start" and put one foot in front of the other. Still others attempt to lift weights but do not fully understand the biomechanics of the various weight training movements or they allow their egos to get ahead of their strength and end up with joint injuries, muscle tears, and tendon issues. And even if a person understands how to lift properly, questions still exist regarding which exercises to perform for which muscle group, as well as attempts to figure out rep ranges, number of sets per exercise, and number of exercises to perform per muscle group. Some of the answers to these questions are dependent upon the purpose behind an individual's decision to lift weights. Is it for a sport-specific performance enhancement, like building endurance in order to participate in a triathlon, or building power and strength for competing at a powerlifting meet, or shaping individual muscle groups and creating size and symmetry for standing on stage at a bodybuilding show, or creating explosiveness for an MMA fight or karate championship? Or is it for personal achievement—never to be used in an athletic- or aesthetic-based event—and what are those personal goals and desires for one's body? Additionally, are there previous injuries or stability and mobility restrictions that must be taken into consideration?

There just is not a one-size-fits-all approach to weightlifting. Garnering help from a professional coach or trainer will provide the most benefit to beginners, intermediates, and advanced athletes alike who wish to learn the proper way of lifting as well as receive guidance on how to work each muscle group and which exercises will enhance performance or shape the muscle to meet one's athletic and/or aesthetic goals. It is best to choose a coach or trainer who carries personal experience within the desired field of sport or competition, the necessary educational qualifications or certifications, as well as has excellent references who can vouch for success with said coach or trainer. Below is a set of questions to run through in order to hire the correct professional for the best end results.

1. What is my end goal? Be sure to return to Chapter 1 if you do not have this in hand already.
2. What type of accountability and motivation do I need? Do I want a professional with whom I may physically visit for check-ins or benchmark measurements as well as training sessions in person? Do I need someone to personally show me how to perform the exercises? Or am I self-motivated and can I search for someone who works in a different city, state, or country, in which the main mode of communication is online?

3. What type of qualifications do I want this person to have? Does a long list of certifications impress me? Or does actual experience within said sport, athletic event, or aesthetic competition matter even more to me? What is the right combination between these two categories?

4. How many and what type of references should I request?

5. What is my budget for this portion of reaching my end goal?

6. How much time am I willing to commit to training? How many days per week and how many minutes or hours per day?

7. Do I want someone contracted to a specific gym? Or would I fit better with an independent contractor who may be able to travel to wherever I am? Do I care or prefer whether I am in a franchise gym, a "Mom and Pop" type of gym, or a private studio? And do I need to be a member of the gym in which this professional coach or trainer works?

8. Should I request a consultation meeting or a trial period to test out the professional before locking myself into a monetary agreement?

9. What are the top three to five most important attributes I wish to see in the professional I plan to hire, and how will I figure out if said professional has those attributes?

10. What type of results do I expect to see in what amount of time frame that hold both myself and the professional coach or trainer accountable and utilizes our time and resources best?

11. What are my deal breakers where this professional is concerned? What would cause me to fire this coach or trainer? And what would cause me to re-hire this person after my initial time frame is up? Am I willing to share both of these pieces of information with the professional right away?

Tools to Assist You

Ultimately, you are the only person who can enlist change in your lifestyle. But positive reinforcement, active support, and constructive criticism are all critical components to ensure a successful journey of change. In turn, your actions will motivate others, creating a very dynamic process of action, compliment, action, correction, action, compliment, action. As you can see, motivation is a bi-directional concept: Perform the action, show the results, trigger motivation in others to enact their own results, take on constructive critiques in order to improve performance, and others learn from your improvements and successes.

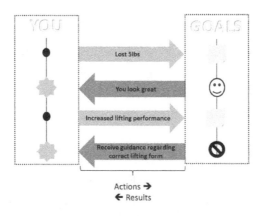

Figure 3-3: The dynamic process of actions

It becomes a partnership in which positive energy, words of encouragement, and visual changes occur for all involved. What may have originally seemed like a deserted-island goal in turn becomes a metropolis of results. Self-confidence then soars to skyscraper heights, creating a true lifestyle change that involves not just the physical self but also the mental and emotional aspects to you as a human being. This is why many of the tools suggested here involve communities of individuals who are just like you: wishing to make a true lifestyle change in a healthy manner. By sharing your daily choices along with documenting your progress, you create an accountability mechanism. Breaking old habits and creating news ones that may appear boring at first or tough and monotonous are definitely challenging actions in life. The beginning stages offer many hiccups, speed bumps, and setbacks. It is not uncommon to stutter start your way through the process, so having others to catch you when you stumble or to help direct your way when you threaten to detour is important.

Online Community Tools

There are many websites available in which you can peruse other people have accomplished or are in the process of accomplishing in terms of body transformations at all stages. One such example is the website: www.bodybuilding.com, which has an annual competition called "90 Days Transformation." This is a perfect spot to visit online in which you can browse through other people's stories, look at their pictures, and say, "Wow! If he or she could do it, I can do it too!" Remember, we talked about positive reinforcement earlier, and the best form of positivity is by looking at how someone else succeeded and utilizing that good energy to push yourself to succeed in your own goals. This is different from looking at others in an envious fashion, where someone uses negative reinforcement, whispering to themselves, "Why can't I be like that?" Instead, these stories and transformation pictures become an outlet of inspiration and motivation, both propellers of helping you become a better you. In fact, you can go right now to bodyspace.bodybuilding.com/ and create your own personal account. Just set up your profile, write your goals, and begin tracking your progress. Figure 3-4 below displays an example of author Yuri's Bodyspace and the customizable information options you have.

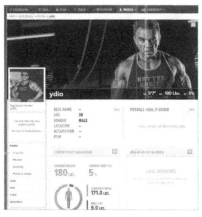

Figure 3-4: Bodyspace from bodybuilding.com
and the options available to customize your plan

If you don't want to create an account, you may still visit www.bodybuilding.com/fun/bbmainmind/transformations. html in order to find some of the transformations that best inspire you. Additionally, bodybuilding.com has an entire network of articles to complement your nutrition and training programs, providing you with a plethora of recipes, food preparation hints, vitamin and supplementation advice, firsthand product reviews, exercise descriptions, and training program examples that help anyone at any stage of their lifestyle change: beginner, intermediate, and advanced.

Another tool you can use to stay motivated as well as share your results with friends and others in the community is Fitocracy: www.fitocracy.com. Featured in a 2012 edition of USA Today[15], this tool is like the Facebook of exercise. In fact, your posts on Fitocracy can actually be integrated with Facebook should you wish to share with your Facebook community as well. Fitocracy also sends out newsletters, provides articles, connects you with others who have similar goals, allows people to cheer you on via virtual sidelines, and gives access to a community of trainers and experts who can help guide you toward your goals in a positive and safe environment.

There are other social media engines that allow you to show off your hard work and browse through others' results. But beware. Technology creates a double-edged sword when it comes to utilizing other people's pictures for personal assessment and motivation. Pictures do not always tell the whole story, especially when access to filters and changes to those pictures is so readily available. Anyone can say anything. Anyone can post anything. It does not necessarily mean it is

---

15   Saltzman, Marc (2012). Fitocracy: A social way to work out. Retrieved from http://content.usatoday.com/communities/technologylive/ post/2012/05/fitocracy-a-social-way-to-work-out/1#.VDVwTvmwnyk

real. And it does not necessarily mean it is helpful. If you use a virtual tool simply for the purpose of comparing other people's results to your own results, then you will quickly drop yourself back to square one in this whole lifestyle change process. You must return to the foundation of your "change pyramid—the psychological aspect and the self-awareness approach. During the moment in which you read stories and view pictures, ask yourself why you are looking at this particular person's information in this particular moment. Determine concretely how this is relevant to your own steps toward improvement. If you cannot answer the why and how, then your time is not being well spent and might actually be counterproductive to your attempts toward success.

The same can be said about what you share. Remind yourself constantly that someone just like you at the beginning of your journey is on the other side of your posts. Less clothing may mean more "likes" in virtual sharing communities like Instagram. But less is not always more. Just like you should ask yourself questions about why you are examining someone else's story and pictures and how those are helping your journey, ask yourself why you are sharing your story and pictures and how this is helping someone else's journey. There is a fine line between creating a community of support and simply garnering for attention from the wrong crowd. Professional bikini competitor in the IFBB (International Federation of Bodybuilding), Nathalia Melo, recently published a picture on her Instagram timeline[16] that shares a great point about women

16   See the picture here http://instagram.com/p/
       s0F9aCBfWN/?modal=true

posting racy "progress pictures" that show more skin for the sake of skin than progress for the sake of progress. A person may be discussing the progress they have made in the growth of their shoulder muscles, but the picture displayed may show everything but the shoulder (i.e., a bikini shot from the top of the chest to the top of the thighs). In essence, inspire others by the following:

1. Your capacity to change,
2. Your ability to align your words with your pictures
3. Your effort to share your experiences, display your results, and teach your lessons learned.

Author, Jodi, has a great example of what a progress picture after a shoulder training session can look like when done appropriately: http://instagram.com/p/paMapzqIWW/?modal=true

Tracking Tools for Nutrition

Regardless of what nutrition program you follow, you should consistently track your caloric intake in order to remain focused with your food choices and to also determine the connection between what you ate and how it affected your body, as discussed in the self-awareness section of this chapter. There are many tools that can help you in this tracking endeavor, with many of them readily available as "apps" for your Smartphone, allowing you to track your nutrition no matter where you are. In order to help you narrows down which tracking tool to use, the following article has a list of the top five tools that will best help your efforts, especially when getting started: http://lifehacker.com/five-best-food-and-nutrition-tracking-tools-1084103754.

MyFitnessPal is one of these tools that we will feature here. Located at www.myfitnesspal.com, this tool allows you to add into the system each item that you ate. It then calculates the macronutrients, as seen in the example below:

Meal 1	Calories	Carbs	Fat	Protein	Sodium	Sugar	
Cochran - Quaker - Instant Grits, Original, 2.5 packet	250	55	0	5	775	0	⊖
0183 Splenda - No Calorie Sweetener Packets, 3 packet (1g)	10	3	0	0	0	3	⊖
Mc - Egg Whites - Egg White, 7 large egg white	119	1	1	25	385	0	⊖
Eggs - Fried (whole egg), 1 large	92	0	7	6	94	0	⊖
Coffee - Brewed from grounds, 1 cup (8 fl oz)	2	0	0	0	5	0	⊖
Add Food Quick Tools	473	59	8	36	1,259	3	

Figure 3-5 Sample breakfast tracked using this tool

If you keep adding your meals throughout the day, the tool will calculate your daily consumption and will automatically compare with your daily goal. At the end of the day, you can check to see if you ate too much or ate just the right amount, as shown below:

	Calories	Carbs	Fat	Protein	Sodium	Sugar
Totals	2,644	254	57	280	1,840	26
Your Daily Goal	2,250	169	75	225	2,500	48
Remaining	-394	-85	18	-55	660	22

Figure 3-6 – Sample of totals where this person
ate more than he or she should have.

Ultimately, this daily reflection on what you are consuming is very important, no matter what your nutrition approach is. In addition to that, study[17] shows that tracking your food intake can help you during the weight loss process.

Finally, this tool can also help you track your weekly or monthly progress using the reports capabilities. Below is a report entitled, "Net Calories Consumed," and it covers one full week, comparing actual calories with the goal for the week. This allows you to look at your progress in a holistic sense to examine where you experience successes versus pitfalls and to compare with other factors in your life that may affect your progress (i.e., work, vacation, illness, etc.)

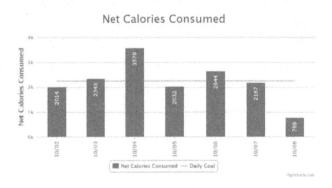

Figure 3-7 – Weekly report of net calories consumed

Tracking Tools for Exercise Programs

Assuming you do have a training program, you can still leverage some online tools and apps to assist you tracking your training. Some people prefer to do this manually, just a notepad with the training and the amount of weight that

---

17   You can find this study in the following link http://www.sciencedaily. com/releases/2008/07/080708080738.htm

they were able to use on each exercise, which works just as well as a technological approach. There is no right or wrong way to track it; you should use whatever works best for you. Some of the tools that I mentioned earlier in this chapter, such as Fitocracy and MyfitnessPal, also have the capability to track exercises and the amount of calories burned. This is a good way to integrate nutrition and calories burned into one application and remain organized.

For people who like running or cycling, there are many tools that can leverage GPS capability to give you precise information about your workout, and the integration of the heart rate monitor will also give an accurate amount of calories burned. One of these tools is the called RunKeeper (runkeeper.com), which is not only for running despite the name. Figure 3-8 below has an example of the interface of this tool:

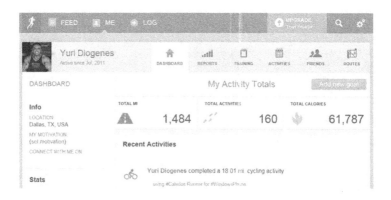

Figure 3-8 – The dashboard of this tool allows you quickly visualize the amount of calories that you burned during your exercise

The one common denominator for all of these tools (for both nutrition and exercise) is the public access they provide. Each one of these tools allows the user to publicly share his or her current status, progress, and goals via numbers and/or pictures. A community of motivation exists in which a person motivates not just him or herself but a whole network of others with similar goals. These tools also provide accountability because, even though it is great to have a training partner and cheerleaders on the virtual sidelines, ultimately, you have to rely upon and push yourself to move closer and closer to your goal.[18]

Wearable Technology

This new category of fitness tools, called "Wearable Technology" moves things to a whole different level as far as monitoring and integration among different tools. Most of them are able to:

1. **Integrate with other nutrition tools:** This is really a great differentiating factor because you will not need to manually add your calories in one tool while tracking the nutrition in another. Basically it saves you time by automatically adding the amount of calories that you burned on that day, which also makes it more precise. For example: the Microsoft Band[19] integrates with MyFitnessPal.

2. **Track your sleeping patterns:** Another very important factor of your daily activities is recovery

18   Read this testimony about be on your own and keep pushing to move on http://instagram.com/p/sAUa59RFjt/?modal=true

19   For more information about the Microsoft Band see http://www. microsoft.com/microsoft-band/en-us

time. If the results of your sleeping patterns tracked by your device, shown that you are not getting enough sleep, you need to rethink your strategy and overall schedule to accommodate a better and longer period of recovery.

3. **Provide real time progress:** Another advantage of many of these devices is the capability of allowing you to instantly show your results, history, and progress. As a matter of fact, the reports that are generated by some of these devices are by far the greatest advantage of having one. Remember: monitoring your results to ensure that you are on track is very important because you can take action based on those results.

It is recommended that you do your own research about the wearable technology that best fits your own needs. Take into consideration those three major components mentioned above, and remember to choose a device that is well integrated with other platforms. When you are selecting a device to assist you in your fitness journey, the last thing you want is to add another layer of concern and or a waste of time; therefore you need a device that will save you time and precisely give you the information that you need about your progress.

Of course, don't forget the importance of purchasing and using a heart rate monitor. It not only allows you to monitor your heart rate, but it also ensures that you are reaching the fat burning zone and safely staying there as much as you can for the duration of exercise. The heart rate monitor can also allow you to take adequate rest in between sets in such way that you don't cool down too much. Be sure to look for heart rate monitors that can be integrated with your mobile app, such as Kyto.[20]

Keep Track of your Results

When we attempt to judge or monitor our own progress with something as subjective as our bodies, we often have difficulties remaining objective without utilizing concrete evidence to mark our results. In Chapter 1, we discussed the importance of setting benchmarks along the way towards reaching our goals. There are many ways to do this when charting our bodies' changes. Unfortunately, simply looking in the mirror each morning is not enough. Below are several recommended tools to rely upon when determining the rate of progress you are making within your fitness journey.

1. **Weight:** When weighing yourself, be sure to do so at the same time of day each time as well as wear the same articles of clothing. A digital scale is often most helpful.

2. **Body Fat Testing:** There are several methods of body fat testing, including calipers, hydrostatic testing, and BodPod testing. All have pros and cons attached to them, so be sure to do your research regarding the person or company administering the test.

3. **Fit of Clothing:** Set aside a particular bikini or set of swimming trunks as well as a pair of jeans that are not too stretchy, and a set of dress pants and button down shirt. Try the articles of clothing on at each benchmark

---

20   More information see http://www.amazon.com/Exercise-Wireless-Monitor-iPhone4S-spinning/dp/B00AW76O1K

period to see how they fit and feel when you stand, walk, and sit.

4. **Progress Pictures:** Take a set of pictures displaying the body from the front, the back, and each side. Be sure to wear the same clothing items (i.e., the same bathing suit or sports bra and shorts set or the same swimming trunks) each time you take pictures. Try taking them at the same time of day as well as in the same spot or with similar lighting in order to retain accuracy of photos. Decide whether you will take pictures weekly, bi-weekly, or monthly.

5. **Measurements:** Use a measuring tape, and have a partner measure the following spots on the body: neck, shoulders, biceps on one arm, chest, waist, hips, thigh on one leg, calf on one leg. Keep track of the measurements and determine how often you will take measurements. Monthly might be a good time frame.

Be aware that playing a numbers game is rarely ever helpful. So be careful when using the first two tools of weight and body fat testing to be the sole determinants of your success. While these numbers can assist you in seeing if you are going in the right direction, they can also trick you in thinking you are worse off than what you actually are. As mentioned earlier, you might be putting on muscle mass while burning off fat; in this respect, the number on the scale is certainly going to rise, but it does not mean you are not meeting your fitness goals. Additionally, there are many factors that affect the numbers when it comes to weight and body fat percentages. Our stress levels, water intake, women's cycles, and time of day—amongst many other factors—can alter the number that pops up. Ultimately, do not over-react or become reliant upon weighing yourself daily or checking body fat and making determinations about your success without also taking into account the other three tools. Finally, understand that your actions ultimately determine the results these tools show back to you. If you are consistent, dedicated, and motivated, you will see results, no matter what method you used to pack your bags for this fitness trip.

Chapter 4
PERFORMING BETTER:
AT WORK AND BEYOND

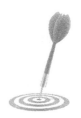

Introduction

Symphonies and songs. Rarely are either of these comprised of just one instrument or just one note. Instead, they are made up of a beautiful blend of the strumming guitar coupled with the deepening bass matched with the beating drum nestled within the lulling voice. When done properly, each musical element ebbs and flows perfectly to create a finished product that makes our ears perk up, our goose bumps rise up, and our hearts fill up. It is the same with the blend of a healthy body partnering with a healthy mind.

Up to this point, we have focused on specific aspects necessary for the process to change your lifestyle. We've examined acquiring mental strength, determining goals, creating plans of action, and setting specific guidelines for individual nutrition and training. And in Chapter 2 we grazed the surface of how your performance at work can be affected when you are in an unbalanced state, much like a broken guitar string or a hoarse voice can throw off the entire song. The intent of this chapter is to go beyond that and to explore in more depth the reasons why a better body equates to a better mind also. You may, by now, already realize that energy will flow much more fluidly and effectively with a healthier lifestyle, but this chapter will discuss how to leverage this energy in the workplace in order to progress further in your professional world.

A Healthy Body Opens the Door for a Productive Mind

According to the CDC (Centers for Disease Control and Prevention)[21]:

> *"Regular physical activity can help keep your thinking, learning, and judgment skills sharp as you age. It can also reduce your risk of depression and may help you sleep better. Research has shown that doing aerobic or a mix of aerobic and muscle-strengthening activities 3 to 5 times a week for 30 to 60 minutes can give you these mental health benefits."*

---

21 Found at: http://www.cdc.gov/physicalactivity/everyone/health/index.html#ImproveMentalHealth

One on One with the Author:
The Side Effects of High Energy
By Yuri Diogenes

In one year's span—from October 2011 to October 2012—I lost a whopping 100lbs[22]. This monumental weight loss was the first phase of my overall change. Just by dropping such a huge percentage of body fat, I noticed an equally enormous gain in energy. I began experience higher quality sleep, which in turn allowed me to wake up earlier due to feeling refreshed from that good night's rest. My mind and body both moved at a faster rate, and I felt I could accomplish many tasks at once, whereas before I moved like a sloth through solitary activities. As a result of this incredible increase in energy, I was able to simultaneously conquer three new challenges: a) working towards a Master's degree, b) writing a new technical book, and c) training for a bodybuilding competition. I did all of this while still working hard in my regular job as well as remaining a conscientious, responsible, and loving husband and father. I had set forth for myself a very ambitious plan that had many spokes in the wheel of my life, and I did this because my main requirement was that I could no longer compromise any area of my life for the sole purpose of succeeding in another area like I had neglectfully and poorly done in the past.

---

22   You can read this blog from Quest Nutrition about this transformation http://blog.questnutrition.com/transformation-tuesday-achieving-the-dream/

I began this parallel journey of training, studying, and writing in November 2012, and I consistently kept moving at a solid, methodical pace through these three goals all the way through June 2014. This juggling act culminated in the following successes: a) I competed at the National Physique Committee's (NPC) Adela Garcia Classic in Pflugerville, Texas, in June 2014. This met my original desire and goal since day one of my weight loss journey: competing in bodybuilding.[23] b) My technical book, regarding Cloud Computing, was released in August 2014 in Brazil,[24] and it sold out in one month. c) During that same month, I also finished my Master of Science in Cybersecurity. Without a doubt, discipline and organization both act as the flutes and trumpets of this well-orchestrated symphony. But that is the thing about succeeding in life: an orchestra doesn't depend upon just one instrument to create a musical masterpiece. Thus, you can achieve many goals within a singular timeframe, rather than just choose mastery in only one area of your life.

Without a shadow of a doubt, I give utmost credit for these accomplishments to my increase in energy level. Good nutrition, solid rest, and consistent physical activity enabled me to achieve these successes as well as focus on my job and maintain a healthy personal relationship with my family without compromising any other areas of my life.

---

23 Here one of the greatest moment of my life at the end of the competition http://instagram.com/p/phus3ORFpv/?modal=true

24 A picture from the book signing session in Recife, Brazil http://instagram.com/p/q63p6SxFvZ/?modal=true

The fact of the matter is: exercise and proper nutrition work wonders for awakening the brain. Ultimately, your mood and aura are positively enhanced. On top of that, your alertness improves, your ability to learn rises, and your productivity level increases.

One on One with the Author:
Fight Depression with Endorphin Elevation
by Jodi Miller

During my sophomore year in college I was diagnosed with depression. Even as an honor roll student in a middle-class family, the signs were all there for the majority of my teenage years: immense fatigue, perennial desire to sleep, vivid mood swings with few catalysts attached, crying spells, thoughts of suicide. The doctor tried to prescribe anti-depressants to me, and I rejected the offer. I instead turned to exercise, both mental and physical, to combat what I refused to alter medically.

Many a morning I would awaken and not want to roll out of bed, not want to start my day, not want to take a shower and pick out clothes and fix my hair and apply my make up and step foot into the open air that existed beyond the confines of the apparent safety of my apartment. During my early twenties, I taught high school English and of course *had* to walk out that door and enter the real world from Monday through Friday. But Saturday and Sunday would arrive, and I would find myself sitting on the living room floor, rocking myself back and forth, immobilized in a despair from which I could not find the beginning or the end, like a tangled ball of yarn. The one thing...the one thing that could draw me out of the dark rabbit hole was the gym. After all, I had goals. Powerlifting goals. Bodybuilding goals. Goals that required a plan of action and steps to take and moments to achieve. One does not acquire a six pack by the wave of a magic wand. Meals have to be prepped and weights have to be lifted and treadmills have to be trekked. It takes weeks and months, consistency and dedication, stubbornness and determination, fortitude and clarity. All things that disappear when depression appears, things that depression steals like a thief in the night. I had to fight through the fog in those moments, pick myself up off the ground, blow my nose, apply a touch of concealer under my bloodshot eyes, throw on gym clothes, and get in the car to drive to the gym. Once in the gym, the weights became my anti-depressant. The heavier the dumbbell and the more weight on the barbell, the lighter the load on my heart. The more sets I completed and the more my muscles burned, the less I ached inside the recesses of my mind. By the time I was done with my workout, a grin cracked my face and I returned to a normal, happier state of mind.

To this day, I still deal with depression. Over 20 years later. And to this day, I rely upon the gym and my goals in powerlifting and bodybuilding to grab me by the hand and yank me out of that rabbit hole. Like taking an Advil and believing your headache will disappear in an hour, I take my dose of exercise and know that within 60 to 90 minutes, I will return to a safe place inside my heart and mind.

Of course, you cannot go out for a run one day, eat a broccoli stalk, and come back the next day having successfully met all of the goals you set forth in your life. There is a progression of energy and skill as well as a process to improving in all areas of your life. And the techniques discussed in Chapters 1 and 2 that are used to accomplish goals for losing weight or gaining strength transfer very well to accomplishing goals in all other sectors of life, including career, education, other hobbies, and family. By following those tactics, you truly gain more time in your day because of the following elements:

- *Self Empowerment*: You no longer linger in bed or think only of the tasks that a boss has set forth for your day. Instead, you take charge of your day from the get go, turning the alarm off instead of tapping snooze multiple times. You step into your day tackling personal goals, which makes you more open to meeting other people's requests, needs, and deadlines. In this way, you add time to your day to meet your goals, whether they relate to your career, your family, or yourself.

- *Organization*: The more regimented you are in your personal life, the more regimented you become in your professional sector. When your day fills up with activities that are constructive, active, and positive, filling out a planner with day's "to do's" becomes a more pleasant experience. Tasks are written down, prioritized, and checked off or transferred to the next day if necessary. Small rocks—as discussed in Franklin Covey's 7 Habits of Highly Effective People—don't clutter the daily jar; instead, big rocks become the main focus.

- *Mental Clarity*: As mentioned earlier, the CDC's website generalizes a correlation between overall mental health and consistent, regular physical activity but does not delve into specifically how physical activity builds mental health. Recent studies, such as one led by the Georgia Institute of Technology, shows that weight training can improve memory.[25] While we might think we don't need our memory banks since our smartphones and laptops and other 21st century gadgets do so much of our remembering for us, in reality we need to keep up with the quickening pace of our technologically-advanced society. Keeping track of professional events, business contacts, personal dates, and general skills needed for our careers, like answering questions on the fly in meetings, is still necessary regardless of how many "smart" devices sit on your desk. Shaping your body essentially shapes your mind and thus shapes the direction of your career achievements.

- *Accomplishment*: Just as organization in one area of life breeds organization in other areas, so does accomplishment. Success becomes contagious. Imagine waking up, drinking your coffee and water, and completing 20 minutes of HIT cardio before ever spooning a bite of oatmeal into your mouth. A goal for the day is ticked off the list, and no matter what

---

25   Read this article for more information on this study: http://www. sciencealert.com.au/news/20140610-26289.html

happens to try to stand in your way, your successful start will certainly breed successes in other areas of your day, like running a web conference for the northwest sales division, teaching a new computer software trick to a co-worker, completing a spreadsheet report, showing a house to a real estate client, etc.

- *Camaraderie*: An old adage states "misery loves company." That is certainly true, but good work ethic also loves a crowd. People, much like cream, rise to the top. By exhibiting in your daily behaviors and rituals small—and large—steps of success, others who are serious about their own intentions of self-improvement will slowly let go of personal excuses and begin to ask you, "How do you do what you do?" See, the only way that your motivation truly serves as a role model quality is if you share what you know and what you do. This means leading by example—as shown in Figure 4-1—being proud (not arrogant) of

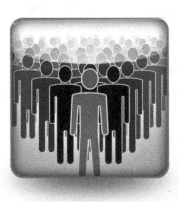

Figure 4-1: Lead by example and have more followers

your body transformation, and ensuring your personal life and your professional life parallel each other by not allowing one to overshadow or deplete the other.

One on One with the Author: Lead to be a Leader
By Yuri Diogenes

In 2012, I led a project that basically started a completely new venture for the Information Technology (IT) community in Brazil. I lived in Texas at the time—as I do now—and as a result, all my interaction and communication with my Brazilian IT cohorts utilized the Internet. However, I had to convince this same community—from a distance—to produce content using a new, virtual platform with which nobody was familiar. Basically, I was asking professionals in my industry to trust a new process that had no preceding reputation or review. Essentially, we would be pioneers.

I decided the best way to start this technological "evangelization" was to personally be the guinea pig and utilize the new platform myself in order to write our technology news articles and then publicize these articles via social networks. I was going out on a limb and trying something that had risk and potential of failure, but I buckled down and got to work anyway. Each day, I produced more and more material until I felt confident enough in bringing my work to the social networks. I then sat back and watched the results. Once I saw the rise in attention to my articles via the social networks, I then requested a meeting with top technical leaders in the Brazilian community. I showed them my articles, the social networks that publicized the articles, and the positive responses from others. I then asked these same leaders to do exactly what I did: take a chance, risk failure, and try a new platform to get technological communication into the public sector.

Management workshops always preach, "lead by example." This is easy to do when a manager demonstrates success within his or her comfort zone. But a true leader demonstrates leadership by stepping outside of that comfort zone, putting in top notch effort, making mistakes, and learning from the mistakes in order to demonstrate improvement. By doing this, that leader opens the door for his or her constituents to do the same within their own roles.

I did this very thing, and afterwards I reaped the rewards when a program manager for the social network platform publicized my efforts in an article entitled, "Yuri is the Shirtless Man." By stripping myself of the cloaking fear of failure, I clothed myself in success, improvement, and confidence.

Visit this link and read the complete article and video that was used as reference: http://blogs.technet.com/b/wikininjas/archive/2012/05/18/brazil-on-technet-wiki-yuri-is-the-shirtless-man.aspx

Beyond Self-Esteem

Many people initially decide to change their body with the hopes of regaining or building self-esteem. There is nothing wrong with that. Low self-esteem coupled with inactivity can actually lead to depression. A new study performed by researchers at Karolinska Institutet in Sweden[26] shows that physical exercise can protect the brain from stress-induced depression. So there is no drawback to beginning a lifestyle change with the initial thought of, "Hey, I just want to look at me in the mirror and feel good again," serving as a catalyst to a perennial change. The fact of the matter is, low self-esteem can spill over into all areas of life, including work, and cause problems due to a poor perception of self and a lack of belief in one's ability to perform.[27]

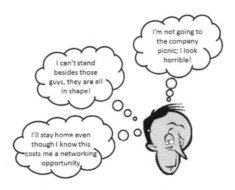

Figure 4-2: What are the excuses that you will come up with because you are not ready to deal with the facts?

But sometimes a person centers attention on the desire to feel better about oneself, and when self-esteem does not skyrocket overnight, motivation and dedication threaten to melt away,

26   More information at http://www.sciencedaily.com/ releases/2014/09/140925131345.htm

27   This article mentions a study that was performed to understand how low self-esteem can cost your job: http://www.forbes.com/2010/07/22/ confidence-job-satisfaction-interview-techniques-forbes-woman-leadership-self-esteem.html

and junk food binging enters the scene. So improving one's self esteem should be an added benefit of the transformation ride or journey, not the whip that beats the horse into a faster race. When this is realized, then it is easier to tiptoe out of one's comfort zone and hop into unfamiliar territory that introduces risks, new skills, possibility for mistakes, and situations for learning. Each day, purposely choose one thing that pushes you outside of that comfort zone. It could be anything like trying a different route to jog in the morning or joining a new recovery yoga class or signing up for an Excel spreadsheet class when normally you would just teach it to yourself. Or you might present a new team management idea to your boss that will help the whole office to succeed, or you might purchase paint supplies from the local hardware store and begin repainting the walls of your abode. No matter what it is, try something new. You might not succeed. The walls might look messy. Your boss might turn down your idea. You might fail the Excel class and not get professional development credit. You might lose your balance in yoga or not come even remotely close to performing the splits. And you might get tired and have to walk the rest of the way home along that new route because you miscalculated distance. But then again, you might learn. And you might do better the second go 'round. And even better, you might succeed. Either way, flip the switch on the fear of failure by facing failure head on and inviting it into your life. When you accept the chance of failure, see it as a learning experience, and allow yourself to take a risk to succeed, you build self-esteem at a quicker rate than if you just go by the book and only do what is expected of you, especially if you are the one setting the original expectation. See, self-esteem and self-confidence are built via all areas of one's life, not just in a superficial, skin-deep sense. Uncovering your six-pack will not always transfer into disseminating your insecurities. Instead, by simultaneously succeeding in tasks and meeting goals in both personal and professional arenas and by finding rewards that are not food-based but instead geared towards self-improvement and endorphin release, confidence increases exponentially. And then you experience a lifestyle change that truly lasts the span of a lifetime.

Shield Yourself at Work

We have spent the majority of this chapter discussing the positives of making a lifestyle change. Many people will applaud you for your efforts, inquire about your strategy, and celebrate your success. But jealousy can often rear its ugly head, and when it happens in the workplace, it can create reverberating consequences that may threaten to set you back to the beginning of your journey.

Shielding Steps

There are many steps you can take to shield yourself from the shrapnel of any sabotage by others surrounding you. Consider the following steps:

1. Become aware of and recognize jealousy; accept the fact that it will occur whether you want it to or not.
   - It has been argued that the way you look can influence how others perceive you and respond

to you. In a study performed in 2011, led by Professor Rosario Zurriaga,[28] women were found more likely to be jealous of a workplace rival if she was attractive. Often times, as we lose weight, build muscle, re-shape our bodies, and essentially transform ourselves, we improve our attractiveness. We also tend to change our hair, wear more form-fitting and currently fashionable clothes. We smile and laugh more, which can be misconstrued as flirtatious behavior. We walk with our shoulders back, our chests high, our chins upright, and that air of confidence adds to the attractive nature. All of these signal a threat to others who may not have tapped into their own self-improvement reservoir. The key is to recognize that our increased attractiveness due to our lifestyle changes may elicit a negative and jealous response from others even if we are minding our own business and not stepping on anyone else's toes. Once we recognize it can and does occur, we can be quicker in accepting it and turning our focus back to our plans of action to change, grow, and challenge ourselves daily.

2. Assess the negative action, realize that you can only change your reaction to others' actions, and do not judge the person performing the sabotage.

---

28   The complete study can be found here http://www.researchgate.net/publication/233844909_Open_Topic_Articles_Gender_Differences_in_the_Jealousy-Evoking_Effect_of_Rival_Characteristics_A_Study_in_Spain_and_Argentina/links/0912f50c0e3a8afc7c000000

- If you focus on the action itself, you deal with a factual circumstance and avoid opinions based upon emotion. When you judge another person for judging your choices, you simply repeat what that person is doing to you. For example, if a person at work always leaves a doughnut on your desk every Monday morning when she brings doughnuts for the entire office even though you have already explained that you do not eat sweets, stop trying to change this individual and instead deal with the doughnut itself. Re-gift it to another co-worker who does enjoy sweets. Transfer the doughnut to the community kitchen. Wrap up the doughnut and give it to the homeless man at the intersection outside your office. Or simply throw the doughnut away later in the day. No matter what, do not eat the doughnut, and do not turn your frustration onto the woman. Ultimately, you cannot change the behavior of this woman leaving the doughnut on your desk. She may very well be sabotaging you. Or she might simply be scatterbrained and never remember you don't eat sweets. Either way, trying to change her actions over and over is like beating your head against a wall in order to move the wall. The doughnut is a much easier object to change and move. And ultimately, weight loss is your battle for which you must take responsibility and action. If you cannot avoid eating a doughnut when it is placed in front of you, then it is time to go back to your original goals, re-examine your motivational mindset, and create a new game plan for when obstacles such as this enter your sight.

3. Learn to understand the root cause of the behavior, but do not expect to change the behavior of anyone but yourself.

- Let's return to the woman leaving the doughnut on your desk every Monday even though you have explained you do not eat sweets. Maybe she just went through a divorce six months ago and has gained 30 pounds due to emotional eating when under duress. Or maybe she had a death in the family and food is her coping mechanism. Or maybe she has diabetes and cannot eat sweets but projects her cravings onto others by buying doughnuts once per week and doling them out like candy on a Halloween night. Or maybe she really does wish to sabotage you because she is truly jealous of your improvements and insecure in her inability to make a change as of yet in her life. You will not be able to *fix* any one of these issues, but by seeing the woman as a human being with feelings and flaws just as you are, you create a connection and understanding that allows you retract anger and resentment that would only fuel the fire of this woman's inability to support your goals. And in turn, you free yourself to turn your focus to your own goals and returning back to step one: dealing with the action at hand rather than trying to change the person doling out the action.

Give to Get: The Act of Mentorship

This last step in the shielding process is a lengthy one but also the most productive and far-reaching one. By acting as a mentor to others and sharing what you know without losing the pre-determined pace you have set forth in your original plan of action, you create a unique sense of wealth that can turn the tides of jealousy in a positive manner. The key is to do this without the expectation that others will change but instead with the sheer desire to share knowledge and let people make their own choices in their own time.

Always remember you do not need to downgrade the level of your service in order to welcome others into your circle of knowledge. You just need to encourage others to perform at a higher level. Many companies have a mentorship program as part of their Human Resources professional development plan. In fact, the companies that do have an official mentorship program linked directly to professional development and career rewards will not only recognize the efforts of the mentor but also the active engagement of the mentee. Mentoring works tremendously because it allows a person to lead by example while adding patience and concrete teaching skills into the mix.

Mentors typically focus their teachings based on their career role, general expertise, and overall education within the company or organization. For example, a software engineer may mentor a newcomer to the engineering department and focus solely upon the software system that this company uses. But a project manager for the same company may mentor the software engineer in learning how to examine a project from a big-picture angle rather than just focusing on software code to get the job done. No matter your role, thinking outside the box in order to draw someone's attention and improve upon his or her skillset is a necessary component to the success of both the mentor and the mentee. Additionally, taking the time to understand the personality, attitude, habits, strengths, and weaknesses that this person brings to the table is essential to ensuring you are working with the current flow of the person and not against his grain.

Part of being a mentor includes creating new initiatives that utilize your knowledge and allow others to work towards their own goals. This means you must understand your colleagues; learn about their interests, their habits, their strengths, and their weaknesses. This requires talking to your colleagues and observing them. For example, you might watch your department over the span of a week. Maybe you notice that no one in the department takes a true lunch break. Instead, everyone works through lunch and then intermittently heads to the vending machine to grab candy bars, peanut butter crackers, and sodas as pick-me-ups in the dead of the afternoon. They then work until 7 or 8 p.m. after having arrived at work as early as 7 a.m., and at least 60% of the department experiences crashes around the mid-afternoon time frame. Productivity becomes slower; chatter between cubicles increases; mistakes pop up in afternoon emails. As a result, you might start an initiative to obtain permission to pull from the petty cash fund, go to a store that sells in bulk or in discount pricing and purchase fresh vegetables, fruits, packages of tuna, and packets of oatmeal as free snacks for the department. Or you might tackle the issue from a different angle, examining the root cause like we discussed earlier in this chapter, and understanding that a work-life balance needs to be set in motion. As a result, talk with the manager of the department about building an acceptance and understanding that breaks from work are necessary, especially to eat. Collaborate with the manager for both of you to lead by example and take your own lunch breaks at least three out of the five work days per week.

Other Best Practices to Turn Negative Behavior from Others into Positive:

Other best practices that go hand in hand with mentorship and can be used to further shield yourself from others' jealousy and even convert it to admiration include the following:

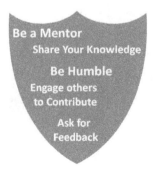

Figure 4-3: Important factors to shield yourself
while empowering others

- **Be humble:** There is no better way to welcome others than by being humble. It doesn't matter if you are on the cover of a magazine or if you won the Nobel Peace Prize. Without humility, your character and value become diminished, and your bulb in the public eye will grow dim.

- **Engage others to contribute:** Rather than engaging only your upper-level managers in conversations and ignoring subordinates in your division, make sure everyone is engaged by speaking equally to all and sharing ideas with all. As you move higher in your position, you cannot forget your roots; your peers are precious assets to you and your genuine appreciation towards them will also help avoid jealous backlashes later in your career.

- **Encourage others to give feedback about you:** Feedback sometimes can be tough, especially when that feedback[29] provides constructive criticism. Rather than letting your emotions lead the way when someone explains how you can improve, instead do the following:
  - ▲ Listen to the feedback.
  - ▲ Repeat with your own words.
  - ▲ Ask for specific examples of the areas needing a fix as well as areas that were done well.
  - ▲ Discuss openly what a successful solution would look like to the person that gave you this feedback.

---

29 Read this article from Harvard Business Review to learn the key questions for effective feedback https://hbr.org/2011/08/three-questions-for-effective-feedback

▲ Determine a plan of action to approach improving the weak areas as well as strengthening the positive areas.

▲ Ask for feedback again once those actions have been completed. All of these steps, when taken appropriately and actively, enable growth and strengthen the overall lifestyle change you initiated in the first place. This process also strengthens the confidence and character of the person providing the feedback to you, especially if this is an upward feedback situation where a subordinate is providing constructive criticism to you as his or her manager. And this too may act as a shield against any jealousy that may arise from those who are struggling to improve within their own paths of life.

• **Help others to succeed:** Even if your company doesn't have a mentorship program or your work/life balance idea discussed earlier didn't work the way you intended, still conduct yourself as a champion for someone in your department. Dedicate yourself to consistently assisting a colleague achieve one of his or her goals. Then continue to follow up and make sure that this person you chose to help is in a better place one year from now.

The best teachers are students, so remember that by learning, shielding, and giving, you grow stronger and more successful in the process.

What's Next?

This is probably the most monumental question when we get ready to close out one chapter of our lives and turn the page to start a new chapter. This is the sign of true progression and growth. An ending means an opening for a new beginning, but before you do that, introspection is paramount. Look back on your journey in order to understand the successes and failures of what you have done thus far. Pinpoint your true accomplishments. Examine your mistakes and determine where you learned from those mistakes and where you still need to improve. Determine your output and ensure your investment was worthwhile. Did you get what you were really looking to achieve and was it worth the effort undertaken? You may not have accomplished everything in exactly the way you pictured when you began this journey, but if you are in a better place now than you were when you set foot on this path of change, and then you have succeeded.

Celebrate that success and be aware of where you had to revise strategies and goals due to unexpected speed bumps that are sure to occur in life. Drawing awareness to your flexibility as your path changed is an important part of your journey. In fact, the fickle corporate environment is a perfect example of how handy flexibility can be. Many times our future is uncertain; even if you are stellar performer, the company that you are working for might change gears to adjust better in the marketplace and an entire organization within the company vanishes. Layoffs or transfers may occur. This is where the flexibility you practiced in your personal plan of action transfers well to your professional world. This way, you can relocate or find a new job with as little stress as possible and can open yourself up to learning and experiencing new environments and skills in order to increase your value and leverage yourself in the work force

Once you identify your new desire and goal—what you wish to accomplish next—and understand the risks and variables involved, it is time to start that next chapter and establish your new plan and begin this process of change and improvement all over again. After all, a true artist does not write one song and call it quits. Guitar riffs change, drums create a different rhythm, voices change, and notes shift. And the artist evolves through it all.

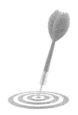

Chapter 5
PLANNING FOR THE FUTURE

Introduction

Take a moment to imagine the following scenario. It is your college graduation day, and you are about to walk across the stage to take ahold of your diploma, move your tassel to the left side of your cap, and trot down the stairs and into the rest of your employed life. What if you were to refuse the diploma? Walk backwards down the stairs you just climbed and continue that backwards shuffle all the way to your first day of your freshman year in college but still carrying all of the knowledge you gained throughout your four (or five) years of education. Seems silly, right? You wouldn't *redo* your collegiate experience, except maybe a party or football game. But seriously, you definitely would not retake that crack-ofdawn macro-economics class with the soft-spoken professor or the business calculus class with the crazy professor who erased formulas as quickly as he wrote them. Not if you passed those classes fair and square, right? You would instead grab that diploma like a dog snatching a treat out of an owner's hands, race down the stairs, and run straight out of the auditorium right into a graduate program or a job or a backpacking trip across Europe. The point is: you would do something that you had not done previously.

So, why treat your fitness venture any differently than your educational venture? This chapter will guide you through determining your future once you've achieved your original fitness goals.

Decisions, Decisions

Have you ever wished your closet had a door to your very own Narnia just like the wardrobe in *The Lion, The Witch, and the Wardrobe*, by C.S. Lewis? A place where you could walk from one reality into another and become an elevated version of yourself (complete with Turkish Delight)? The process of changing our bodies and changing our minds actually acts like that very doorway into a magical world. Where we once were stale, bored, sluggish, depressed, weak, and weighed down, we now have the power to switch all of these negative qualities into positive ones, and that experience truly is magical and breathtaking. The key is ensuring we do not return to that original state from which we came. And that can only be achieved if we choose to continue to elevate ourselves, to create more magic, to challenge ourselves, and to take ourselves to the next level.

One on One with the Author: What to do Now
by Jodi Miller

At the ripe old age of 18, I essentially began my weightlifting career as a powerlifter. The person who took me under his wing on the very first day that I entered the free-weight room was a national collegiate champion powerlifter, so all of my training, technique, and form were based upon powerlifting principles. Though I had only done two meets within the first five years of my weightlifting experience, I had personally prepped as though I was doing meets each year. Once I turned 24, I began to step away from powerlifting. My coach at the time suggested I take time away from the sport and instead just simply work out. He wanted to make sure I was in the weight room to lift weights because I truly loved the iron and not just because of my seemingly intrinsic competitive spirit. After two years passed, I decided lifting weights for giggles was not enough, and I began to search for a competitive outlet.

At the time (and this will age me incredibly), the bodybuilding world only had two divisions: fitness and bodybuilding. There was no "figure" nor "physique" (men's or women's) nor "bikini" (except those seedy bar contests). My options were incredibly limited. But I continued to search and research. I thumbed through magazines such as *Oxygen* and *Ironman*. I perused ESPN on early Saturday mornings. I talked to people in the gym. It was actually the glossy pages of *Oxygen* that presented my little Narnia to me: obstacle course competitions. At the time, the

Galaxy and Women's Tri-Fitness were two organizations that offered an alternative to fitness and bodybuilding competitions for those who had no gymnastics background or those who did have enough muscle mass for the stage. These obstacle course competitions required the hundreds of female competitors to run a military-style obstacle course on the first day of the competition and then come back the next day in a bikini and heels to display on a spotlighted stage an athletic physique. Jackpot!

The only trouble? I was petrified of heights, and the Galaxy Federation required competitors to climb up a 15-foot high cargo net and flip over to the other side and scale downward to the ground before running to a 10-foot high rope wall, pulling oneself up to the top, flipping to the other side, letting go, and landing on the ground. When I say "petrified" of heights, I mean to the point of hyperventilation on high bridges when driving and fear of escalators. I had it bad. But I was determined to face my fears and compete.

I did just that, and I am so glad I didn't just continue in the weight room for giggles. Two years later, I had moved on from the Galaxy Federation into the National Physique Committee (NPC) shows, winning my first ever bodybuilding show with a routine done to Destiny Child's *Bootylicious* (yes, I'm a tad bit embarrassed and yet proud at the same time). The point is, nothing that I have accomplished in these past 24 years would have occurred if I twiddled my thumbs, allowed my fitness venture to stagnate, and accepted status quo for myself. No Ms. Natural Olympia title. No NPC Team Universe win. No venture back into powerlifting to earn a

World Championship qualification and decimate any previous records or personal bests I had set in earlier years. No risks. No mistakes. No lessons. No Jodi as I am known today.

I couldn't imagine that, and so I'm glad that I have a spirit that requires forward movement even in unfamiliar territory. It keeps me young at heart.

There really is a method to the madness of choosing an unchartered path. And it really is as simple (and hopefully less ironic) as Robert Frost's poem, "The Road Not Taken." All it takes is laying out all of your options—even farfetched ones—just like laying out all of your clothes for the suitcase you'll take on a trip and then researching each option. Then choosing the one that best fits you, even if it is a "road not taken" by anyone else you know in your own inner circle.

The following steps will help you configure your future and guide you away from the auto-pilot whirlpool that so many get caught up in because they don't know what steps to take or are too scared to take any steps into deeper waters.

Lists

We make lists for tasks of the day, groceries to buy, errands to run, gifts to get. We sometimes forget that personal lists are just as important as material lists. Your first list should be about the things that you are good at and that you like to do. See an example of such a list below:

- Hiking
- Reading

- Staying regimented
- Being outdoors
- Lifting weight (a lot of weight)
- Teaching
- Traveling
- Having alone time

Don't rush through the list. Take a few days to write it up so you can make sure you capture all of your qualities and enjoyments.

Common Thread

Look at the items on the list and determine a common thread through the majority of the qualities. What is that one bright blue thread that pops up through the entire sweater of your internal make up? Write it down in the margin of your list. If we return to the sample list above, one common thread might be that almost all of the items can be accomplished alone, without the aid of others.

More Lists

Now, write a list of all of the activities, events, competitions, hobbies, etc., that utilize your best qualities, likes, and attributes as well as allow this one common thread would to serve as an attribute. Below is a brief example:

- Powerlifting
- Bodybuilding
- Mountain hiking

- Triathlon

There is actually a plethora of activities, events, competitions, and hobbies in which to partake in addition to the ones already mentioned:

- Strongman
- Olympic lifting
- Mixed martial arts
- Gymnastics
- Dance (of all variations)
- Skiing (water or snow)
- Marathons
- 5Ks
- Decathlons
- Spartan races
- Tough mudders
- Crossfit
- All categories of bodybuilding (including bikini, fitness, figure, physique—men and women)
- Charity walks
- Fun runs
- Team/intramural sports (volleyball, softball, hockey, basketball, etc.)
- Golf

Research

This step is actually one that can be started prior to making a list of all the activities or events you should consider partaking.

Some research must be done to see what is actually out there and available for the taking. After you compile a list of activities and competitions, then you return to the research step and begin determining everything that is involved with each hobby, activity, event, or competition in which you are interested. Below are the categories to research and their subcategories or explanations.

- Fees/Monies
  - ▲ Determine all of the things you need to purchase and how much each item will cost. This includes clothes, suits, shoes, joining fees, travel fees, activity fees, coaching fees, etc.
  - ▲ Compare this with your own budget to ensure this hobby will fit with your current lifestyle and management of living expenses.
- Organizations to join
  - ▲ Most organizations require their participants to join yearly.
  - ▲ Clothes and shoes required
  - ▲ Do you need a swimsuit or swim trunks? If so, what do they need to look like? Can you purchase these from the store or online, or do you need the outfit specially made for you?
  - ▲ Do you need heels or tennis shoes or other foot attire?
  - ▲ Do you need specific clothes like a wrestling singlet or baggy pants or t-shirt with sleeves of a specific length?

- ▲ Do you need jewelry? Do you need to remove jewelry (i.e., navel adornment)?
- Overall appearance
  - ▲ For women, do you need to prepare hair, make up, and nails for a specific look or presentation?
  - ▲ Is a tan required?
- Level of competition
  - ▲ What level of experience is needed for this competition or event?
  - ▲ Is it a starter/beginner event, a national qualifier, a pro qualifier?
  - ▲ Are there age groups? Weight requirements Height divisions?
- Previous competition or activity results
  - ▲ What are the winning times from previous events?
  - ▲ What are the winning weight totals from previous events?
  - ▲ What are the skills utilized by the winners?
  - ▲ What do previous winners look like? And non-winners?
    - ○ Peruse pictures to see what separates first place from second place and so on.
    - ○ Peruse pictures to determine where you might fit in right now and later at your best. This better ensures you are choosing the right division, hobby, or event.
- Location(s) of events
  - ▲ In the same city?
  - ▲ In the same state?

- ▲ In the same country?
- ▲ Would you drive or fly to the event? Do you need a hotel room? Do you need a kitchen?
- ▲ What transportation do you need once there?
- Time involved for the event
  - ▲ Is it just a few hours? A day? Several days?
- Time involved for the preparation
  - ▲ How many days, weeks, months, or years do you need to begin advance preparation for weight lifting programs or nutritional changes?
- Finding experts and facilities to support and guide you
  - ▲ What type of coach or trainer do you need?
  - ▲ What credentials do you want this coach or trainer to have in regards to the skill in which they are teaching you? (I.e., experience versus certification)
  - ▲ How often do you need to visit or work with this coach/trainer?
  - ▲ Are there classes you need to attend to learn the skill?
  - ▲ Do you need to join a particular gym or have access to a particular setting like a stadium or track or hills or trails or swimming pool?
  - ▲ Are there other competitors in your area or online who have done this activity recently who can guide you?
  - ▲ Are there online resources you can use (social media, forums, articles, etc.)

Moment of Truth

You have done the grunt work. Now it is time to face reality and couple it with your desire to reach a new goal. Do you have what it takes: the grit, determination, funds, time, and resources? What often helps is creating a T-chart that lists out pros and cons of incorporating a goal of this magnitude into your life. On one side, write up all of the positives that will come out of working towards and attaining said goal. On the other side, write up all of the drawbacks. Compare the two columns and determine if you are ready to take a step into your own Narnia and elevate yourself into a new level of your life.

As you know, life is a cycle . . . ever changing. Temperatures drop. Leaves fall. Branches are left bare and shivering in the cold of winter. Temperatures rise. Buds bloom. Branches are weighted down with fresh greenery. Roots expand. Growth occurs. And so you too will do the same and return right back to the beginning in which you fish for your dream, capture it with the bait of knowledge, and bring it to fruition via everything you have learned here.

Those waters are plentiful. Don't ever stop fishing. Don't ever stop dreaming. Don't ever stop achieving.

ABOUT THE AUTHORS

Yuri Diogenes, MS, MBA, technical speaker, NPC competitor based in DFW Texas and author of more than ten technical books published worldwide. Yuri started his lifestyle change in 2011 and in the first year he lost 100 pounds by following a specific nutrition, training program and by changing his mindset to focus on the balance approach in life. It is this balanced approach that he will describe in this book. You can follow Yuri Diogenes on Twitter @yuridiogenes and on Instagram @ydiogenes.

Jodi Leigh Miller is a graduate from The University of Texas at Austin with a BA in English and a lifetime secondary teaching certification in the state of Texas for grades 6 through 12.

Jodi taught ninth-grade English for six years and later became an instructional leader, having trained and managed new teachers in the educational reform organization, The New Teacher Project. Jodi has competed in multiple divisions of the bodybuilding industry, including Figure, Women's Physique, and Bodybuilding. She won the lightweight bodybuilding division of the 2007 NPC Team Universe and participated in the IFBB World Championships in Spain later that same year. She earned the Ms. Natural Olympia title as a professional competitor in the PNBA organization in 2011 and 2012. She has also broken state and national powerlifting records in the APF and competed in the 2014 WPC World Championships, where she set new world records for her division. She is also a top-five, national-level NPC Women's Physique competitor. While her background is in education, she is currently a personal trainer and a competition posing coach at …destination Gym in Plano, Texas. You can follow Jodi Miller on Instagram @jodileigh, on Facebook www.facebook.com/JodiLeighProAthlete, and on Twitter @jodileigh2128.